Medicine in Old Age

For Churchill Livingstone:

Publisher: Timothy Horne
Project Editor: Barbara Simmons
Copy-editor: Wendy Lee
Project controller: Nancy Arnott
Design direction: Erik Bigland
Artist: Ethan Danielson

For information on Churchill Livingstone titles, or to place an order, call:

UK: Freephone 0500 566 242
Europe: +44 131 535 1021
USA/Canada: +1 201 319 9800
Australia/New Zealand: +61 3 9699 5400

Medicine in Old Age

S. C. Allen BSc MD FRCP (Edinburgh and London) MBA

Consultant Physician in General Medicine and Geriatric Medicine, The Royal Bournemouth and Christchurch Hospitals, Dorset; Honorary Clinical Teacher, Southampton Medical School, Southampton

FOURTH EDITION

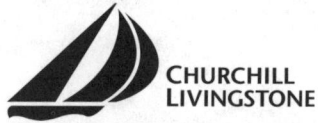
CHURCHILL
LIVINGSTONE

EDINBURGH LONDON MADRID MELBOURNE NEW YORK SAN FRANCISCO AND TOKYO 1998

CHURCHILL LIVINGSTONE
Medical Division of Pearson Profession Limited

Distributed in the United States of America by Churchill
Livingstone Inc., 650 Avenue of the Americas, New York,
N.Y. 10011, and by associated companies, branches and
representatives throughout the world.

First edition 1976
Second edition 1981
Third edition 1987
Fourth edition 1998

ISBN 0443 057788

British Library of Cataloguing in Publication Data
A catalogue record for this book is available from the British
Library.

Library of Congress Cataloging in Publication Data
A catalog record for this book is available from the Library
of Congress.

Medical knowledge is constantly changing. As information
becomes available, changes in treatment, procedures,
equipment and the use of drugs become necessary. The
author and publisher have, as far as it is possible, taken care
to ensure that the information given in the text is accurate
and up-to-date. However, readers are strongly advised to
confirm that the information, especially with regard to drug
usage, complies with current legislation and standard of
practice.

Produced by Longman Asia Ltd, Hong Kong
NPC/01

Preface

This book was originally conceived and written by Professor J C Brocklehurst and Dr T Hanley from the University of Manchester Department of Geriatric Medicine in 1976. At that time it was the first book of its kind and became popular with medical students in Britain and overseas. I joined the authorship in 1987 when Dr Hanley retired and Professor Brocklehurst and I wrote the third edition. There have been a great number of developments in geriatric medicine in the intervening ten years, so for this fourth edition I have completely rewritten the book and it has been laid out and presented in a more modern style. Nevertheless, the purpose of the book remains the same as when it was first published; that is, to introduce medical students and other healthcare professionals in training to the particular problems of medicine in elderly people, with special emphasis on the main clinical presentations such as falls, incontinence, mental confusion, immobility and social breakdown. I have added a new chapter on respiratory disease in old age, since this is an extremely important and prevalent cause of morbidity and mortality. I have also introduced a separate chapter on rehabilitation.

The book does not set out to be a comprehensive textbook of geriatric medicine; indeed, there are a number of excellent major textbooks in that field. Also, I have not provided comprehensive guidelines to therapy, the details of which are also dealt with thoroughly in a variety of other publications.

Geriatric medicine and gerontology are now firmly established in the undergraduate curriculum of virtually all medical schools in the United Kingdom and in a great many in other parts of the world. The subject is now an important part of the final examination for medical students and forms an important component of the MRCP examination for postgraduates. Furthermore, as the population becomes more aged in the United Kingdom and similar countries, the need for doctors to have a thorough understanding of the medical problems of old age has never been more important.

I hope, therefore, that this book will introduce young healthcare professionals to the essentials of dealing with medical problems in elderly people which will stand them in good stead in their professional practice and examinations

I would like to record my thanks to my fellow consultants at the Royal Bournemouth Hospital, Dr M Z K Rana, Dr D Jenkinson and Dr K Amar. The frequent and lively discussions on all aspect of geriatric medicine which take place in our department have formed an important background to the style of practice represented in this book. I also wish to thank Lisa Anzinger-Cooper for her immaculate typing of the manuscript, and Barbara Simmons of Churchill Livingstone and Wendy Lee for their invaluable advice on the final production of the book.

Bournemouth, 1998   S C A

Contents

Part I

Ageing and old age

Theories on the nature of ageing

The science of ageing has grown enormously in recent years. Much research is under way, and our understanding of the biological process of ageing is advancing slowly. Nevertheless, there is no one unifying theory of ageing which is accepted by all gerontologists; consequently, theories have proliferated. That humans should be fascinated and preoccupied with the concept of ageing is understandable, since we are the only living creatures capable of grasping it as an idea and consequently of fearing it and wishing to understand or even control it.

Though none of the current theories of ageing can give us a full explanation and understanding of the process, some of the more credible ones, discussed below, can help us to understand at least part of the process and thereby form a basis for further enquiry and research. By reading this chapter the student will be introduced to some of the more important theories of ageing, a grasp of which is important in the practice of medicine, particularly in old age.

A definition of ageing

Like the theories of ageing, there are many definitions of ageing, but one which has stood the test of time and science is that suggested by Alex Comfort which states that 'ageing is characterized by failure to maintain homeostasis under conditions of physiological stress, a failure which is associated with a decrease in viability and an increase in vulnerability of the individual.' For complex organisms such as humans, three important facts about biological ageing should be borne in mind:

1. It is universal – it affects everybody.

2. It is deteriorative – diminishing the function of cells and therefore organs and the organism.
3. It does not cause breakdown in homeostasis until ageing changes become extreme, or until the system as a whole is stressed. The amount of stress required to cause a breakdown in homeostasis falls as a system becomes more aged.

An example is ageing in the cardiorespiratory system, which does not impair the normal old person's ability to move around and perform normal activities of life. However, if the cardiorespiratory system is stressed, by running to catch a bus for instance, it will fail sooner than that of a younger person. This particular example will be enlarged on in later chapters of this book but the general principle can be applied to any physiological system.

The major theories of ageing

There is still a tendency for ageing theories to be polarized into those which are known as programme theories of ageing and those generally described as error theories.

In the former it is contended that the entire process of ageing is genetically encoded and that progressive expression of the appropriate genes throughout life leads to the changes of ageing and ultimately to death of the organism.

On the other hand, error theories contend that environmental influences on the organism lead to errors in gene transcription and protein synthesis, and that the steady accumulation of these errors is the cause of ageing and death. The vast majority of individual theories of ageing fall more or less into one or the other of these broad categories, though a more sophisticated view is now emerging which suggests that ageing is both programmed and the result of error; thus the two theories are not necessarily mutually exclusive. In the paragraphs below these concepts are enlarged upon to shed some light on the scientific background and the importance of these theories in clinical practice.

A machine analogy of ageing

The human organism can be regarded as a kind of machine, awesome in its complexity and durability but nevertheless doomed to suffer the fate of all machines which are regularly used.

Sooner or later they develop faults, wear out and eventually cease to function, unless there is a sufficient programme of servicing and replacement. Pursuing this analogy, one can deduce some principles that might apply to biological ageing, such as:

1. Deterioration of a machine that is at all complex will occur at several levels of organization. At the lowest level there is an inevitable deterioration with passing time of the basic materials, analogous with metal fatigue or the decay of wood. At a higher level of organization there could be failure of a component with a specific function, e.g. the spark plug of an internal combustion engine; or there could be failure of a system such as the electrical supply which services many components.

These three kinds of machine ageing would roughly correspond with three levels of human ageing: in cells, in organs and in tissues such as blood.

2. The more complex the machine, the greater the likelihood that faults will appear; they will be of different kinds, have various degrees of importance for the function of the machine as a whole, and will evolve at different rates.

The machine will develop increasing numbers of faults with time and will need to be replaced by a completely new machine of the same type. This is broadly analogous to the reproduction of complex organisms.

Although there are clearly many facets to the process of ageing it is rational to look for one or a few processes that could be the common denominator.

It seems logical that the mechanisms of biological ageing should involve the same special properties that distinguish living things from non-living objects. Two basic properties are:

1. the capacity to reproduce
2. the ability to draw energy from the external environment and marshal its use in an orderly way.

Both these unique abilities of living organisms depend on the capacity to synthesize proteins. The physical form of an individual is determined by structural proteins, and the main components of the biochemical machinery concerned with energy production, the enzymes, are also proteins.

Another unique and remarkable property of living tissue is that it has, within the nuclei of its cells, a message in code which gives exact instructions for the synthesis of all proteins in the body.

It is, therefore, not surprising that many of the more important current theories of ageing focus on this coded system of protein manufacture as the most likely place for the passage of time to exert its effect. However, as mentioned above, the manner in which ageing influences protein synthesis is seen differently by the two broad schools of thought in the theory of ageing. These are:

1. Error theories – with deterioration of the protein-synthesizing machinery.
2. Programme theories – the continued operation of a programme which starts as embryonic development, continues as growth and differentiation, and terminates as senescence. This is sometimes referred to as the molecular clock hypothesis.

Error theories

We will now consider error theories of ageing in more detail.

Ageing theories based on deterioration of the protein-synthesizing mechanism

The process of protein synthesis can be distilled into the following succinct phrase:

DNA makes RNA, and RNA makes protein.

Two main subtheories of ageing concern these individual steps:

- That based on abnormalities of 'DNA makes RNA' is commonly called the primary area hypothesis.
- That concerned with 'RNA makes protein' is called the non-DNA error theory.

Most students will be familiar with the basic concepts of DNA transcription and protein synthesis, which can be summarized as follows: the coded message giving instructions for protein synthesis is written along the length of one strand of the double helix of DNA contained in the cell nucleus.

The code is written in terms of the special surface shapes and charge of the four base substances: adenine (A), cytosine (C), guanine (G) and thymine (T). The coded message consists of a particular sequence of these base substances with each amino acid being coded by a unique triplet, e.g. GGA codes for proline.

The message is written on only one strand of DNA: this single strand has to be made available by unwinding of the double helix, and it has to be unbroken to be perfectly comprehensible when decoded.

The DNA letters A and T can behave like lock and key, as can C and G, but no other pairs are possible. The lock and key effect depends on a strict stereochemical fit of the two molecules. The complementary pairs, one member on each of the DNA strands, are responsible for holding together the strands of the double helix.

The first step in decoding is to prepare a complementary copy of DNA message as a long chain of RNA in which uracil (U) replaces T. The process is called transcription and the transcribed copy is messenger RNA, a large molecule located in the cell sap at special assembly points called ribosomes. Below is an example of how a sequence of three DNA triplets is transcribed into messenger RNA:

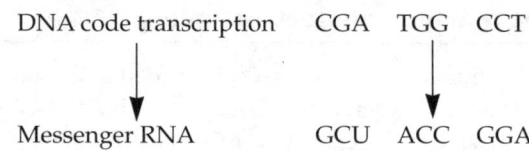

DNA code transcription   CGA TGG CCT

Messenger RNA   GCU ACC GGA

Three basic rules apply:

1. The code is in triplets; each triplet specifies one particular amino acid.
2. It is read in one particular direction.
3. The starting point for reading out must be identified.

In the hypothetical example given above, the protein assembly would occur as follows:

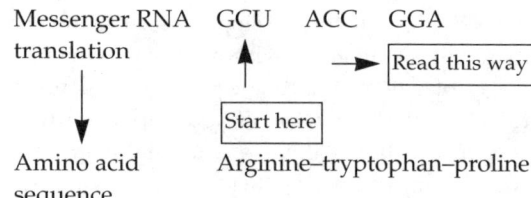

Messenger RNA translation   GCU   ACC   GGA

Read this way

Start here

Amino acid sequence   Arginine–tryptophan–proline

Each amino acid concerned is carried to the construction site on small transport RNA molecules specifically designed to carry that particular amino acid. The transport RNA for a particular amino acid has a complementary anticodon which keys into the messenger RNA lock and so locates the amino acid when its code comes up on messenger RNA. This is an extremely simplified version of the process; in reality, a fairly small protein will contain about 300 amino acid units, and many structural proteins and enzymes contain thousands of amino acids.

Primary error theories – based on disturbances of 'DNA makes RNA'

Most primary error theories are concerned with the possible ways in which the coded information on

DNA could be distorted. This is summarized in Figure 1.1. In the text that follows, capital letters in parentheses refer to Figure 1.1.

Errors of manufacture of DNA (A). This occurs through faulty synthesis or through mistakes during the repair of broken or damaged DNA **(B)**, leading in cells capable of dividing to a mutation, which can be perpetuated indefinitely. In cells incapable of dividing **(C)**, the error cannot be passed on to the next generation but in both kinds of cell the ultimate effects on DNA damage are expressed as:

1. death of a cell **(D)**
2. no effect **(E)**
3. nonexpression or unwanted expression of a gene **(F)**

4. synthesis of wrong molecules or of an altered level of the correct molecule **(G)**.

Damage to completed DNA. This can occur through various mechanisms, some of which are described as follows:

1. *Deformation of the DNA bases themselves.* The free radical theory suggests that oxidative changes in DNA make some of the letters of the code unrecognizable. The evidence for this comes from the hastening of ageing by radiation and by the effects of certain chemicals which induce mutations.

The attraction of the theory lies in the fact that antioxidants exist which protect against radiation effects; this offers a possibility of verifying the

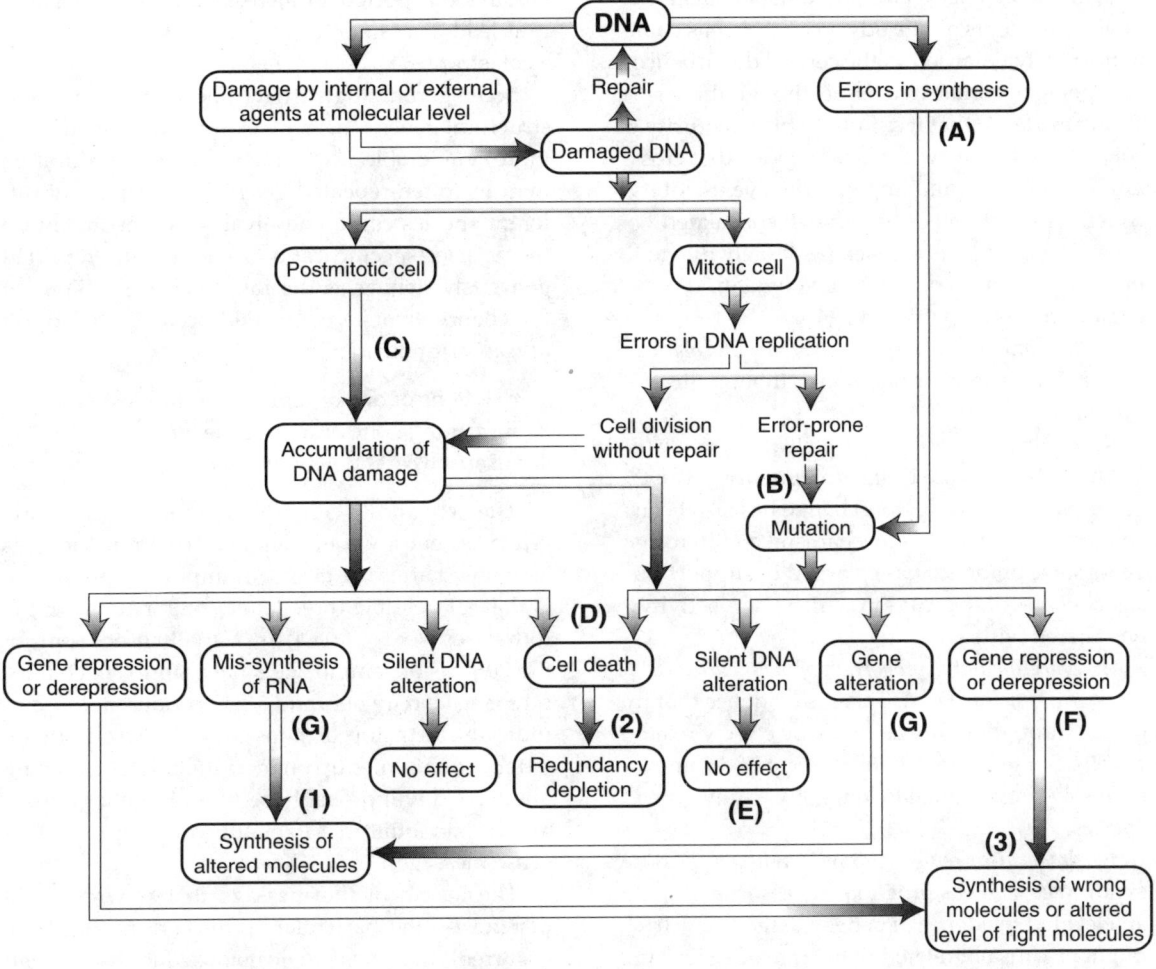

Fig. 1.1 The results of damage to, or errors in, synthesis of DNA.

theory experimentally and there is some evidence that, in huge doses, ageing may be slowed. The difficulty of the theory lies in finding the likely source of either intrinsic or extrinsic DNA damage in natural ageing. The most natural source of mutations is cosmic ionizing radiation.

The effect would be expected to consist of a series of random hits affecting one cell at a time and producing different DNA abnormalities in each nucleus which is hit, but calculation of the probability of hits on DNA from this source makes it highly unlikely that extrinsically induced mutation is a significant factor in ageing. Furthermore, the prevalence of genetic abnormalities in man could not be accounted for by known extrinsic factors.

2. *Changes in the cross-linkage of DNA.* It is known that increased cross-linking of collagen molecules occurs as age advances. This has come to be widely regarded as the central disturbance in the ageing of connective tissue, though there is strong evidence that it simply implies maturity of collagen and not true ageing. The idea that cross-linking in DNA could impede effective use of its coded information has been much speculated upon, but solid facts are lacking, largely due to the immense technical difficulty involved in comparing young with old DNA.

3. *Irreparable breakages in the DNA information strand.* This is another possibility, though direct proof is not available.

4. *A change in the capacity of DNA to react with histones.* Histones are basic proteins which can cover part of the code; this change has also been suggested as an ageing mechanism, and in recent years some evidence has emerged to support this as being one of the ways in which DNA activity has altered with age.

5. *A decline in the proportion of methylated cytosine in nuclear DNA.* There is evidence that this occurs throughout life and may be closely related to cell ageing. Furthermore, the rate of decline is inversely proportional to longevity in any given species.

6. *Premature ageing syndromes in humans.* These syndromes, such as progeria, are associated with an elevated incidence of genetic defects which might be causally related to the rate of ageing in such people.

It is likely that these changes at DNA level will contribute at least something to the phenotype of ageing in humans, though the gathering evidence would suggest the accumulation of genetic defects may be just one of many causes of ageing.

The random error hypothesis

Much attention has been paid to the possibility of random error in the transcription and translation processes described above. A particular hypothesis, the error catastrophe hypothesis, proposes that errors occur in the machinery for making enzymes and more especially in those enzymes (polymerases) which are themselves involved in transcribing DNA. Transcription by a faulty enzyme would be expected to increase errors further and thus lead to a self-accelerating effect culminating in a catastrophe.

Some gerontologists have speculated that those structural genes which are expressed only once are more vulnerable to random error deterioration than the often-repeated genes: the lifespans of different species could conceivably be dependent on the species-specific ratio of unique to repeated genes (shortening as the ratio increases). Some of the chance errors which could occur in the course of transcription are:

1. deletions of one or more code letters
2. insertion of one or more code letters
3. insertions and deletions combined.

The chemical consequence of transcription errors is that a wrong sequence of amino acids is assembled after the error. An important point here is that all possible three-letter combinations of the four bases ($4 \times 4 \times 4 = 64$) are actually used. Some of the 20 possible amino acids have up to six codons, others have only one, and a few codons are used to indicate start, stop or nonsense. If a wrong three-letter codon comes up on messenger RNA, a wrong amino acid will probably be fitted in, though there are certain built-in safeguards to suppress nonsense messages.

The length of the message that is wrong will depend on the particular coding errors that have occurred. The physiological consequences depend on whether or not any of the amino acid sequences occur in those parts of the protein with functional importance, e.g. the active site on an enzyme.

Auto-immunity in relation to ageing

This is an error theory based on DNA mutation. It is proposed that the lymphocytes, the wandering cells which keep up a vigilant surveyance of what is self and what is not, are also capable of somatic mutation and that this will modify their antigenic properties.

The result could be widespread antigen–antibody reaction in different tissues. Proponents of this hypothesis suggest that ageing effects will be shown by cumulative low-grade histoincompatibility reaction in many tissues.

One piece of indirect evidence for this is the increasing prevalence of various types of auto-antibody in elderly people, though it must be emphasized that this association should not be seen as proof that the theory is correct.

Programme theories

In the preceding paragraphs we have discussed the effects of errors in molecular machinery of cells. We will now examine some aspects of the programme theories of ageing. It has also been suggested that one factor in ageing might be changes in the management information contained in DNA. Such management is achieved by substances, probably basic histone proteins, which by the extent to which they cover DNA decide whether or not the activity of the particular gene will be expressed.

The process of growth and differentiation is a genetic programme in which certain genes are switched on and off in particular cells by molecular clocks of some kind. Within this general framework several quite distinctive ideas are put forward:

1. Ageing is simply a continuation of the programme of differentiation, with death as the last item on it.
2. Ageing has an evolutionary value for long-term survival of the species.

This could be achieved by one of the following mechanisms:

- By positive selection of genes which enter the programme, and which are switched on only after maturity has been achieved. There is, however, no convincing evidence that programmed ageing has in general any advantage for survival of the species. Those who argue against this hypothesis would point out that elephants in the wild usually die because they have ground their teeth flat, and

many predators die from lack of effective teeth and claws.

Death from old age, as we think of it in human terms, is probably an exceptional event in wild animals in their natural environment, so programmed senescence could have relatively little effect on selection of value since it is usually outpaced by other extrinsic causes of death.

- By selection of genes which are an advantage in survival to maturity, but prove disadvantageous later, particularly if they promote reproduction but ensure death.

The disposable soma theory

This theory has evolved out of the concept expressed in the last paragraph, and has gained considerable credence as a teleological theory of ageing based on an interpretation of the molecular clock hypothesis as it applies to a species and the survival of species-specific DNA.

It is not purely a programme theory of ageing because it originated from a molecular theory about the stability of protein synthesis and how this has evolved.

Broadly, the disposable soma theory concludes that organisms have evolved an optimal level of accuracy in protein synthesis, compatible with continued survival, but not overdependent on elaborate energy-consuming proofreading or correction devices; therefore, there is a given probability that errors will increase to a level that will eventually kill the individual.

The trade-off is that enormous amounts of energy are concentrated on reproducing DNA to an extremely high level of accuracy to enable successful reproduction to take place and therefore guarantee the survival of the species. Looked at from another point of view, the theory contends that to achieve maximum reproductive fitness, the optimum investment in maintenance results in finite survival. Conversely, the investment required for infinite survival, that is, an immortal phenotype, will reduce reproductive fitness and thus lead to extinction.

Two other experimental findings are important in relation to the molecular clock hypothesis:

- Firstly, the observation that some cell cultures, normally capable of only a limited lifespan, can transform to immortal cells when they are infected by certain kinds of RNA virus, e.g. the Rous sarcoma virus and Rauscher mouse leukaemia virus.

  The normal sequence of events, 'DNA makes RNA and RNA makes protein', is probably capable of being reversed under such circumstances, with RNA making DNA in the infected cells and the abnormal DNA coming to usurp the normal genetic programme and thus not being subject to the restraints that ageing genes would normally exert on the cell. This observation broadly supports the concept of genetically programmed ageing.
- Secondly, another important finding is the Hayflick phenomenon. Human embryonic lung fibroblasts grown in culture are capable of only about 50 doublings, after which they die. Cells taken from adult lungs die after fewer doubling – for each 10-year span of chronological age, one doubling is lost. This finding could be explained by the presence of a molecular clock capable of counting nuclear doublings. (The clock could not have simply counted elapsed time, because the fibroblast cultures could be held for long periods in the frozen state midway in the experiment, and when unfrozen they assumed their doubling behaviour as though nothing had happened.)

However, the cells showed chromosomal abnormalities at the end of the doubling period so the span could be limited by accumulation of errors in DNA rather than by expression of lifespan-limiting genes.

Summary

In this chapter we have introduced the reader to some of the most important main theories of ageing. Our overall understanding of this field is advancing quickly, and most gerontologists with an open mind and an objective view of the evidence are beginning to conclude that genetically determined factors, random errors and environmental influences will be shown to be important in the overall determination of lifespan.

2

Sociological and psychological gerontology

As the science of gerontology has developed, sociologists and psychologists have made great contributions to the study of ageing and many people from both disciplines now work exclusively in the gerontological field. The social gerontologist is concerned firstly with defining and describing the ageing population, and secondly in considering the problems which an ageing society poses, and the possible solutions to these. Psychologists on the other hand approach ageing in three ways:

- firstly, in developing tests of mental and intellectual function which may be used to measure the effects of ageing on these functions
- secondly, to consider the experience of old people themselves, their desires and their problems
- thirdly, to consider the attitudes of the rest of society towards old people and the reasons for these attitudes.

Social gerontology

Throughout the world different societies have their own approach to the concept of ageing, but many industrialized countries with advanced systems share a good deal of common ground, both in the problems created by an ageing population and in the solutions to these problems.

The general shape of the population structure in the United Kingdom over the last 100 years is shown in Figure 2.1. A very similar change in shape would be seen for other countries of a similar level of industrial and social development such as the Netherlands, Denmark, the United States and Japan. It can be seen that around the year 1900, such societies had a roughly pyramidal structure as far as age groups are concerned, with those in the first 15 years of life being by far the largest numerically. This shape has gradually changed to become increasingly square, and if current trends continue and the proportion of the very old in these societies continues to expand, the population structure will take on the shape of an hour glass, as shown in

Figure 2.2. As would be expected, life expectancy figures through the 20th century have shown a corresponding change, as illustrated in Table 2.1. There are a number of important reasons for this change:

1. the improvement in hygiene and nutrition in such societies
2. an increase in the use of methods of birth control
3. the conquest of certain infectious diseases, by the provision of clean water, vaccination, antibiotics and other antibacterial treatments.

Therefore, whereas tuberculosis was the commonest cause of death in young adults at the beginning of this century in the United Kingdom, it is now a relatively negligible cause of death at any age. Similarly, diseases such as diphtheria, the complications of measles, scarlet fever, meningitis and puerperal fever can no longer be regarded as of major significance as causes of death in rich devel-

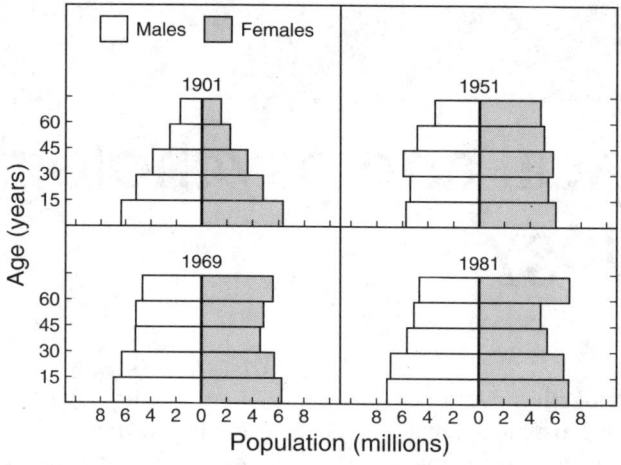

Fig. 2.1 Changes in the population structure from 1901 to 1981.

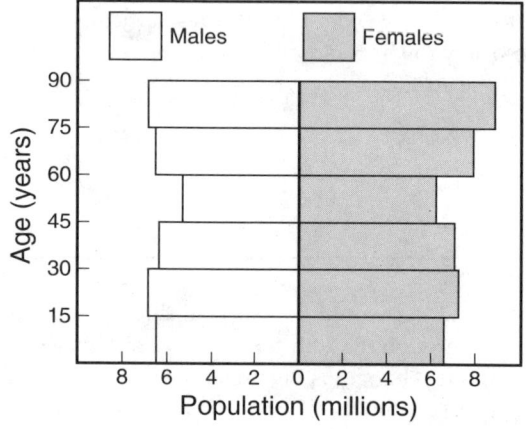

Fig. 2.2 Probable population structure in the UK in the year 2020.

Table 2.1 Life expectancy of men and women at birth and at age 70 in 1901, 1976 and 1986.

Year	1901	1976	1986
At birth			
Male	48.1	69.7	72.2
Female	57.8	75.8	78.4
At age 70			
Male	8.4	9.5	10.0
Female	9.2	12.8	13.5

oped countries. As a result, most people now survive into the years of retirement in those countries and the indications are that as time goes by we shall all live longer periods of our life in retirement.

The ageing population in developing countries

Some developing countries, generally the poorest, have high birth rates, high infant mortality rates and a low life expectancy. Consequently, their population structure is much the same as that in the developed world 100 years ago: that is, very much weighted towards the lower age groups. Some societies have developed very rapidly in the last 25–30 years and thus have unusual population structures characterized by a low birth rate but with relatively few people in the over-65 age band. A good example of this would be Singapore.

Indeed, some of the emerging nations in Africa, and South and Central America have rapidly expanding populations due to the combination of a high birth rate and a rapid improvement in life expectancy. Examples would include Kenya and Mexico. In such countries the proportion of people over the age of 65 is not changing much but the total numbers in that age group are rising rapidly.

Table 2.2 compares the proportion of the population over 65 in 1985 with that predicted for 2005. When interpreting this table some of the changes in

Table 2.2 Percentage of population over the age of 65 in various countries in 1985 and 2005.

Country	% of population aged 65+	
	1985	2005
United Kingdom	15.8	17.0
Canada	10.4	12.5
Japan	10.0	16.5
India	4.3	6.1
Kenya	2.1	2.1
Mexico	3.5	4.6

overall population mentioned above must be taken into account.

Retirement, age and frailty

While the years of retirement are often regarded as being synonymous with old age, this of course is not the case and it is mainly beyond the age of 75 and particularly 85 that the frailty and dependency of chronic illness and of age become apparent. Furthermore, as a result of better living standards, health education and medical intervention, the proportion of people reaching old age in relatively good health is increasing.

This is illustrated in Figures 2.3 and 2.4 which show the changes in the survival and morbidity curves at different times in the 20th century.

Apart from the obvious implication that in the future retirement and old age are going to be the common experience of all of us in developed countries, the most important economic consideration is the fact that the very old are the major consumers of social and medical services. In 1986 the population in the United Kingdom included two people who were either below school-leaving age or retired to every three adults in the working population. As a result of the fall in the birth rate from around 2.5 in 1960 to 1.9 in 1996, the population structure will change so that by around 2010, three people in the population will be dependent on two working, with obvious implications for the economy and planning of services. This problem will not be confined to rich, developed countries, and a rapidly rising number of frail elderly patients in countries such as Kenya and Zimbabwe has already started to raise questions about how to plan for a future which includes a large proportion of frail elderly people, particularly since traditional reliance on the extended family to provide care has already begun to change with increased industrialization, geographical mobility and expectations.

Where retired people live

In all parts of the world the vast majority of elderly people live in their own homes, either alone or with relatives. With increasing age and frailty living alone or with a frail spouse becomes more and more difficult and it becomes necessary for a frail elderly person to receive additional support, often from statutory services, to live alone or to move into some form of residential accommodation. In the United Kingdom about 95% of people over the age of 65 live in private or rented accommodation. Most commonly they are owner-occupiers or living with relatives or friends. Some opt to live in hotels

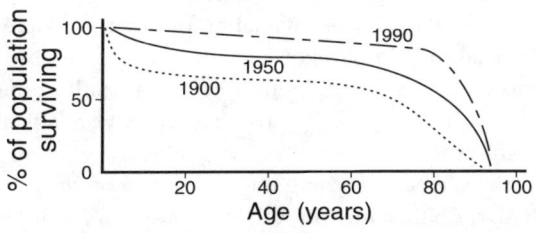

Fig. 2.3 Survival curves for 1900, 1950 and 1990 in a typical old developed country such as the United Kingdom.

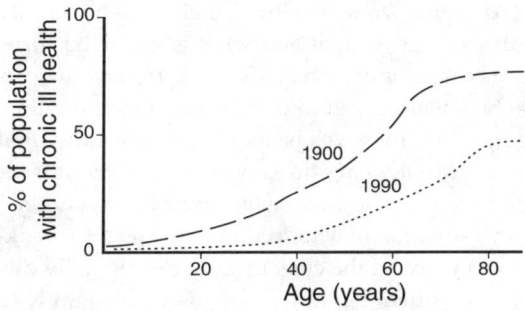

Fig. 2.4 The proportion of the population with chronic ill health in 1900 and 1990 (based on estimations).

or boarding houses and only about 5% live in rest homes, nursing homes or long-stay hospitals. Despite the great expansion in the availability of private-sector rest homes and nursing homes in the United Kingdom in the last 15 years, the majority of residents in such places would previously have been in local authority old people's homes or long-stay geriatric hospitals; thus the overall proportion of people in institutional care has not changed a great deal in that time.

Indeed, the proportion of elderly people living in residential care institutions in the United Kingdom is substantially lower than in most other Western countries; for instance, the proportion is around 8% in Scandinavia and Denmark, 12% in Canada and 7% in the United States of America.

On the other hand, in countries where extended family networks have not been disrupted by geographical, economic and cultural changes, this proportion is generally lower than 5%, even in those with advanced economies such as Singapore, Hong Kong and South Korea.

The prevailing attitude to residential care in the United Kingdom has two important implications. In the first place there is little doubt that most elderly people would prefer to live independently in the community for as long as they possibly can, and that any form of institutional care is the last thing they would wish for or indeed should be encouraged to wish for.

On the other hand, there is no doubt that a proportion of younger members of the population in the United Kingdom are suffering almost intolerable stresses, mental and physical, in trying to cope with aged disabled relatives, especially those who are mentally disordered.

An aged woman with dementia, who hardly realizes what is night and what is day, who turns on gas taps and forgets about them, and who is likely to wander out into the streets in the daytime and get lost, may well be more than any individual person should have to cope with for months or years on end. The stress which may be engendered in this situation may indeed not only lead to breakdown involving the chief carer of the mentally disordered patient but also cause the whole family to suffer.

In view of the extent of chronic brain failure,

estimated to be present in moderate or severe form in up to 8% of people over 65, it may be argued that the figure of 5% institutionalized old people in the United Kingdom signifies greater hardship in this sense than is apparent in other countries.

Family contacts

Surveys indicate that in the United Kingdom people who have children retain fairly close contact with them, though geographical mobility is tending to diminish such contact. Figures for the United States of America are similar to those for the United Kingdom, and in other parts of the world the pattern will be determined by local cultural, economic and geographical factors.

Maintaining contact with children, of course, is not necessarily the same as receiving companionship from them, since it is possible for an elderly person to live in a son's or daughter's house and be almost a stranger, confined to a single room with little contact with other people. However, this is exceptional and while very often old people will maintain a strong determination not to impose any load on their children by going to live with them, it seems to be the case that the majority of widows and widowers with surviving children do have reasonable contact with them.

Major upheavals such as the First World War also have an effect. Until recently a large number of elderly women in Europe were childless as a result of losing husbands and fiancés in the First World War. This generation has now largely died, though small family size during the depression of the 1930s still has some effect and the elderly generation who lost spouses in the Second World War also constitutes a relatively lonely group. In other parts of the world, disasters of a different nature are having an effect on the support available for elderly people. For example, in parts of Uganda a very large proportion of young adults has died as a result of the AIDS pandemic, often leaving elderly relatives unsupported.

Decisions concerning the future way of life, particularly either moving into a residential home or moving to live with the family, should as far as possible never be taken at a time of crisis, such as immediately after a bereavement. The family physician should be able and willing to advise on these matters, if only to do no more than indicate the various possible pathways that are open and the risks and advantages of each.

Loneliness

It is often said that loneliness is the scourge of old age. Inevitably at a time when a spouse is lost and when other friends and contemporaries are dying, and when this is associated also with increasing infirmity, perhaps limited mobility and sensory deprivation such as deafness, loneliness can only be expected to become more common than at younger ages. It is important not to confuse loneliness with being alone. Many people live alone quite happily and others can be lonely in a crowd. There can be little doubt that loneliness is a real problem among elderly people and it is here that the voluntary organizations have more to offer perhaps than any other in providing friendly visitors and the whole network of clubs and day centres, together with some assistance with transport to get there.

The general practitioner should be fully aware of voluntary services that are available in the locality and what they can provide. Family doctors also have a role in stimulating the voluntary organizations to discover the gaps in their services and to attempt to fill these.

Retirement migration

The elderly population in the United Kingdom is unevenly spread. For many years, but particularly during the 1960s and 1970s, people tended to retire to holiday resorts and so areas such as the south coast, the North Wales coast and the main holiday towns in the North-west and North-east of England

have a resident population which contains an exceptionally high proportion of aged people. Some examples are shown in Table 2.3. In some retirement towns there is uneven distribution of the elderly population within that town. For example, there are districts of Bournemouth and towns along the Hampshire coast with as much as 45% of the population over the age of 65, with very large numbers in the over-85 age band. This patchy distribution can cause problems for local family doctors who carry an excessive number of very frail old people on their lists.

In some parts of the United States quite large communities have developed where almost all the residents are retired, with examples in Florida, Arizona and California.

Nevertheless, such phenomena are the exception and in most parts of the world old people live alongside younger members of society and are fairly evenly distributed, though in some countries where industrial development has led to migration of young people to towns, as in parts of South and Central America and South Africa, there is a relatively higher proportion of elderly people in the rural areas.

Table 2.3 Proportion of the population over the age of 65 in various towns in the United Kingdom

Town	% of population aged 65+
Bournemouth	27
Highcliffe-on-Sea	42
Torbay	34
Eastbourne	36
Colwyn Bay	35
Milton Keynes	18
Luton	15
National average	**17**

The psychology of ageing

This has become a very large branch of psychology with much research currently being undertaken, particularly in the United Kingdom, Europe, North America and Japan. The various psychological tests can be useful tools, both in research and in the management of patients. The details of such psychological tests are outside the scope of this book but the student needs to bear in mind that these are available and may be useful to indicate impairment of intellectual function and give some indication also of the prognosis in relation to brain disease in old age.

Recent research has shown that psychological tests and psychometric tests to determine cognitive function, executive function, anxiety and depression can be very useful in assessing potential benefit from rehabilitation in old age, and in tracking the psychological response to that type of approach to treatment.

Old people's attitude towards ageing

One view of the psychological changes with age suggests that old people tend to develop one of two attitudes towards ageing, these being:

1. *Body-transcending*. The elderly person is accepting and realistic about the biological effects of ageing and tends to concentrate on intellectual activity, relationships and the spiritual life.

2. *Body preoccupation*. The old person is highly aware of the deterioration which occurs with senescence, resents this and worries about it, and spends much time thinking about health and disease. Some develop morbid hypochondriasis.

Of course, these two stereotypes are extremes and many people will lie somewhere along a spectrum between the two. Furthermore body preoccupation is not the same as a healthy lifestyle which could include many elements which are beneficial physically, such as exercise, healthy eating and a sensible use of health services. Leisure and comfort may mean predominantly physical well-being and to such a person, the increase in frailty which accompanies age may be hard to bear. On the other hand, others suffer severe pain and discomfort, but

for them social and mental sources of pleasure and self-respect transcend the discomfort. It seems likely that these attitudes to ageing are extensions of a person's personality in younger life. In general it seems that the very old living in the community form an élite who are optimistic about health, seem to have a high social conscience and maintain high spirits.

In fact it has been shown that most old people think their own health is at least as good as, if not better than, that of their contemporaries.

Some elderly people gradually disengage themselves from the social environment, and this is in keeping with the sociological theory of disengagement which was prevalent in the 1960s. However, it is now generally accepted that most old people maintain a very high level of social involvement and activity and that this forms an important ingredient of successful ageing. Indeed, there is a welcome and increasing trend for old people to become involved in educational activity, widening their intellectual experience and exploring ideas which are quite new to them. Further education classes cater for such people in a variety of ways in many societies in different parts of the world and many are able to take distance learning degree courses with organizations such as the Open University. Research now suggests that disengagement may be appropriate to the very last stages of life, perhaps weeks or months. This occurs in the absence of complicating serious disease and may be a completely normal preparation for death.

Psychological accompaniments of ageing

A number of age-associated factors which are measurable relate to the psychologist's view of ageing. For instance, reaction time is slowed and in the face of this an old person is unable to retain both speed and accuracy. This is one of the reasons why older workers find it impossible to keep up with the pace of conveyor belts in manufacturing and is one of the biological reasons why retirement becomes necessary for many people.

Memory

It seems that long-term memory, particularly memory of the very distant past, is retained throughout life. However, as people age the ability to commit new material to memory diminishes and the old person is seen therefore to dwell more and more in the past. Perhaps these postulated changes in the function of memory are more apparent than real. Memory consists of committing new facts by a process of retention and this requires a number of other attributes.

For instance, the desire must be strong enough to memorize the new material and this involves motivation. Once a career has passed such motivation may wane, as may volition and drive. Similarly, there must be a high degree of interest in the matter being committed to memory.

If memory tends to fail for whatever reason with advancing age, then the older person is at a disadvantage in a technological society where the experience accumulated over a number of years may become obsolete and new techniques have to be mastered.

The advantage which the old person has is in accumulated experience and in wisdom. These, however, are often less relevant in our type of society than in earlier ones where the pace of technological change was slower. One of the fruits of this is that some old people accept opportunities which only occur later in life, such as the writing of memoirs and textbooks, an interest in history, and indeed an interest in old age itself. The older person may of course have an accumulated experience in the manipulation of society and be familiar with its social machinery, such as committees, rules, rituals and other procedures.

These are more likely to be of advantage in positions within the establishment than to workers in factories. They are also of great advantage in many developing countries where village elders still retain considerable power to dictate, shape and arbitrate within their sphere of influence.

Stereotypes of psychological ageing

Various studies on the psychology of ageing have resulted in a number of views and theories which differentiate the ways an elderly person reacts to senescence. Perhaps one of the most durable studies is the one outlined below, though it must be borne in mind that this remains an oversimplification of what happens in reality and individual elderly people may exhibit more than one of the characteristics listed in Box 2.1. As in most studies it was found that these stereotypes are generally continuations of the individual's early life characteristics and, as such, are therefore predictable to a certain extent.

Box 2.1 Characteristics of stereotypes

- *Constructiveness.* These well-integrated people enjoy life and its relationships, and are humorous, tolerant, flexible and self-aware. Such people have usually had a happy childhood and successful continuity in life history. They accept the fact of old age, retirement and death, retain the capacity to enjoy food, work, drink, play and sex, and look back with few regrets whilst looking forward to what is yet to come.
- *Dependency.* These people adopt a socially acceptable but passive role. They are usually unambitious people with fairly good insight. There is a tendency for them to be overoptimistic and impractical. In the case of men they often married late and tend to be dominated by their wife.

  Such individuals are glad to retire, they eat and drink too much, gamble and enjoy holidays. They tend to derive no enjoyment from such work as they may have to do.
- *Defensiveness.* These people characteristically have a stable occupational history, are well-adjusted and socially active, and have always planned ahead and refused help. They are often emotionally somewhat overcontrolled, conventional and habit-bound, and may be compulsively active. They tend to be afraid of old age and to put off retirement, as they see few advantages in it and tend to ignore the prospect.

  (Contd)

> **Box 2.1 Characteristics of stereotypes (contd)**
>
> - *Hostility.* These people tend to blame circumstances or other people for their failures. They are generally complaining, aggressive and suspicious, and often have an unstable occupational history with a tendency to be incompetent in a number of minor ways. They see nothing good in old age, are afraid of death, envy the young and tend to plunge into active work to defer the evil day.
> - *Self-hate.* Such people are critical and contemptuous of themselves, are unambitious and have led a life marked by social and economic decline. They are often unhappily married with few hobbies and tend to feel themselves victims of circumstances. They generally accept the fact of ageing, are not envious of the young, are prone to depression and often look forward to the blessed relief of death.

The study outlined above was carried out on elderly men, but subsequent work has shown that these broad characteristics can also be applied to elderly women and can serve as a general guide to the psychological adjustments to ageing.

Retirement

Retirement is such a crucial accompaniment of ageing in Western and other industrial advanced societies that it requires careful consideration by doctors. The physician should understand something of the problems and implications of retirement, recognize it as a possible ingredient in a number of illnesses and be in a position to advise about how retirement should be approached.

Retirement is a new phenomenon inasmuch as in the second half of the 20th century, for the first time, almost everyone is going to spend a significant number of years living in retirement. Retirement can, and indeed should, be a time of fulfilment when the elderly worker is at last released from toil which may not have been congenial and is free to enjoy the other things in life which was not possible while working. This is the ideal picture and there is no doubt that for many people, it is the actuality.

More often than not, however, it is the person who has enjoyed work who will also enjoy retirement, and those who found work a drudgery often find retirement a time of tedium. Retirement is inevitably associated with a number of types of loss.

1. *Loss of finance.* Most people will be significantly poorer after retirement than before and those who depend on state retirement pensions will find that they have an income which is barely enough to live on. In Europe, North America and Australasia many people have occupational pensions which can be quite substantial, and in some industrially advanced societies with minimal state welfare, such as Singapore, people often set aside considerable savings for their old age. Most poor developing countries are not able to offer their aged citizens any pensions.

2. *Loss of status.* A person's position in the world is frequently judged by his or her work. Thus the day before retirement he or she may be the bank manager, the school teacher, the foreman in a factory or a railway guard. The day after retirement there is a tendency to be labelled an old age pensioner.

Such a transition involves a considerable and usually unlooked-for change in status. A trend towards part-time working in the years following retirement from full-time work is now beginning in a number of societies, so the transition is much less abrupt than it would have been in the 1960s or 1970s. Nevertheless, a significant loss of professional status is often suffered by people at the time of retirement.

3. *Loss of companionship.* For most people their work is the place where they have most human contact. Indeed, for the majority of people in our industrial society it is the principal social organization that they belong to. When they stop work they also lose this large element of companionship and social intercourse.

4. *Loss of orderly and purposeful occupation.* However much people may like or dislike their

occupation, there is no doubt that the routine involved is something by which most of them have come to live. This is perhaps the easiest thing to replace, but such replacement does not always happen.

These are probably the most important losses on retirement and perhaps their particular hazard lies in the fact that generally they assail the pensioner rather suddenly and without there having been any time to take steps to prepare. With the increased availability of leisure and with increased education all round, people are beginning to be better able to cope with the bonus years which retirement brings. Unstable occupation in many European countries in the late 1980s and 1990s has in many cases given people a foretaste of the type of adaptation which will be required at the time of retirement. Furthermore, a large number of people are now able to undergo some form of preparation leading up to retirement which can help to prevent some of the medical and psychological problems which occur upon abrupt retirement from full-time working.

Environment

Finally, in considering social and psychological ageing, it is worth recording that environment inevitably contributes to the success or failure of this process.

Physical design of the space in which elderly people live, the fact that they should be safe and secure without being segregated, that shops and public buildings should be easily accessible and indeed that shopkeepers and public servants should recognize the special needs of the old, particularly those living by themselves, are important.

In some societies a large proportion of elderly people have their own transport but a large number also depend on public transport to maintain their mobility, and this needs to be taken into account in vehicle design and public transport scheduling.

3

Aged patients

In societies with reasonable health infrastructures, old age is the period of life which makes greatest demands on medical services. Furthermore, as the population ages, particularly as the proportion of very old people rises, the proportion of hospital beds occupied by people in the retirement age group rises steeply. Also, as medical technology has increased the range of investigations and treatments available, the expectations of old people, their relatives and their general practitioners for intervention by the hospital service in acute illness in old age have risen very rapidly in the United Kingdom, North America and other technologically developed parts of the world. Indeed, whereas about 40% of hospital beds were occupied at any one time by people aged over 65 in 1980, this proportion has now risen to about 75% in an average district general hospital in the United Kingdom. There has been a corresponding rise in the number of contacts between old people and their general practitioners.

The reasons for these changes can be understood more clearly when a number of important characteristics of disease in the elderly are borne in mind. Listed below are some of the key factors:

1. Some changes affect almost everybody who lives long enough and can therefore be regarded as changes due to ageing and not due to disease. The changes in the cardiorespiratory system outlined later in this chapter are typical of this process.

2. There are many chronic and disabling conditions which people accumulate in the course of their lives and which once acquired are never lost. Good examples would be emphysema or osteoarthrosis.

3. Many old people live in very precarious social circumstances, and these are prone to break down if a further burden of acute illness or disability is added.

4. Because of the effect of the ageing process on physiological reserves, and due to the accumulation of degenerative conditions like atherosclerosis, old people are more susceptible to acute illness than other groups of the population. Therefore, stroke, myocardial infarction and pneumonia are examples of common conditions which are found much more often in old people than in the young.

All these factors indicate both the human and the economic importance of dealing with illness in old people in a thorough and competent manner.

It is sometimes argued that when people are approaching the end of their lives medical treatment is less relevant and investigation may therefore be justifiably less thorough. The very opposite, however, is the case because almost all disease processes can be ameliorated in elderly people and some can be cured. Unless the initial examination is thorough some important aspect of the spectrum of disability may be overlooked and the last years of an old person's life may be unnecessarily dependent on others.

Because disease in old age is so complex and because its concomitant disabilities may so affect the life not only of the patient but also of the family and society at large in which the patients lives, there is every reason why medical examination and assessments should be just as meticulous at this age as at any other.

When does old age begin?

Biological and chronological age do not perfectly coincide. Some people show signs of an advanced age in their sixties while others reach their eighties with only modest declines in their physiological reserves.

Too much attention, therefore, must not be paid to chronological age, although there are usually obvious differences between people in their sixties and those in their nineties.

Economic circumstances and factors such as nutrition probably also play a part in this, so that in affluent societies such as Western Europe, North America and Japan, a large number of people reach their late seventies before they start to show real signs of old age.

Those unfortunate enough to suffer from the deprivations of famine, war or excessive manual labour can appear to have many of the physical characteristics of old age by the age of 55 or even earlier.

Geriatric patients

The effect of ageing

The general background of age-related changes which inevitably occur has a limiting effect on a number of bodily functions. For example, changes in the lens lead to presbyopia, changes in the cochlea lead to presbyacusis and a reduction in the accuracy of maintaining posture increases the amount of sway in the standing position. This is illustrated in Figure 3.1.

Details of the changes that occur in the respiratory and cardiac systems are given in chapters 13 and 17, though Figure 3.2 illustrates the overall effect of age on maximum oxygen consumption during exercise which can be seen as an index of the performance of the cardiorespiratory system as a whole. These changes will occur with age to a greater or lesser extent irrespective of the general health of the individual and by the time extreme old age is reached, obvious age-related changes will be seen in all physiological systems.

Accumulated disease

It is not always easy to distinguish between the changes which are attributable to age and those which are due to disease. An example of this is the condition of osteoporosis, important because it predisposes to bone fracture. Osteoporosis is generally regarded as an age-associated disease which is particularly severe in postmenopausal women. However, it is also known that a number of pathological conditions can predispose to or accelerate the development of osteoporosis, such as pro-

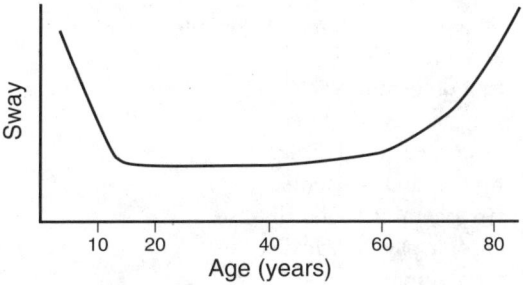

Fig. 3.1 Sway in the upright position rises steeply in old age as posture-maintaining mechanisms age.

longed immobility, poor nutrition, excess alcohol intake or corticosteroid treatment.

Therefore, there is an element of ageing and an element of superimposed pathology in the genesis of osteoporosis. Similarly, atherosclerosis is undoubtedly a disease process, though in Northern Europe and North America there are few who escape its effect as they grow old.

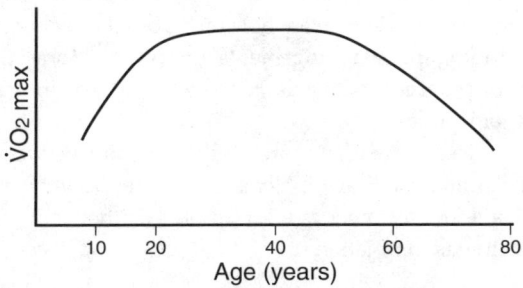

Fig. 3.2 The maximum achievable oxygen uptake during exercise ($\dot{V}O_2$ max) inevitably declines in old age, even in the fittest individuals.

Other examples include impairment of the control of body temperature which is partly due to age-related changes in the hypothalamus but may be made worse by cerebrovascular disease or dementing processes such as Alzheimer's disease. Again, a tendency to postural hypotension in old age may be partly related to ageing in the autonomic nervous system although it is often also partly due to specific autonomic neuropathies in people with, for example, diabetes mellitus or Parkinson's disease. Drug therapy may also make postural hypotension worse.

Other common conditions which result in accumulation of pathology include:

- Osteoarthrosis
- degenerative disease of the intervertebral discs and spondylosis
- foot deformities
- chronic lung disease
- cerebral arterial disease
- myocardial ischaemia
- peripheral vascular disease
- chronic psychiatric disorders
- renal impairment.

This list is by no means exhaustive but does represent a large proportion of the accumulated pathology seen in old patients.

Precarious social circumstances

Many old people throughout the world live in circumstances which are socially very precarious for one reason or another. For example, they may be entirely dependent on a spouse or sibling, or as a result of retirement and bereavement they may be isolated.

Because of physical and mental disability they may be dependent on a whole range of social services including special arrangements for housing, domestic help, provision of meals, home nursing and many other services.

Indeed, there is far more likely to be a link between social and medical problems in old people than in people of any other age group and neither may be dealt with in isolation.

Iatrogenic disease

Old people are often made ill or have their disease

processes complicated by medical treatment. This affects an increasingly significant proportion of the very old, partly because multiple pathology leads to multiple prescribing, and partly because of impaired compliance, with the patient taking more or less than that which is prescribed. Also, the pharmacodynamic changes of old age make some patients particularly susceptible to the side-effects of certain drugs.

The effect of an acute illness

When an aged person with advanced age-related changes and possibly accumulated chronic pathology, who is living in social circumstances which are only just about supportive, has an acute illness, this tips the balance towards social breakdown and often leads to an acute problem requiring immediate attention by medical and social services. Similarly, sudden loss of social support, such as the death of a spouse or other carer, can have the same effect.

An acute medical illness may be so dramatic that it would lead to a hospital admission in a patient of any age, such as myocardial infarction, cerebral haemorrhage or septicaemia, but in very aged and frail people, relatively minor acute medical conditions such as a deep venous thrombosis or ascending urinary tract infection may necessitate admission to hospital, when in a young person the same condition could be treated at home.

Memory

It is often assumed that aged people have impaired memory. Of course, people with a definite dementing disease will have severe impairment of short-term memory and this is relatively easy to demonstrate and measure. However, evidence from recent research suggests that in healthy old people the ability to lay down new memory is very well preserved providing sensory functions are in good condition and motivation is high. Only in extreme old age does significant memory impairment become part of the normal ageing process. The following key points are important:

- Older people can still learn new skills with practice.

- On testing of straightforward mental tasks, the performance between different age groups is trivial.

- Very old individuals are able to improve their mental task performance by practising.

History and examination

Illness in old age is extremely complex. The history and clinical examination must therefore discover not only the final and precipitating factor which has actually brought the patient to a doctor, but also the other diagnoses, and so, adding them all together, the nature of the total illness.

For practical purposes, indeed, it is better to think in terms of problems than of diagnostic labels. The problems are those things which make it difficult for the old patient to live independently in a community. These are functional difficulties.

A hemiplegia, for instance, may have very different implications as far as future lifestyle is concerned for an elderly man living with his younger and able-bodied wife, and for an aged spinster without relatives living entirely alone. Thus, while a full list of diagnoses should always be made at the end of the examination, the problems should also be listed.

The geriatric giants

Irrespective of the underlying disease processes and diagnoses there are five major problems which are often presenting symptoms of illness in old age. These have come to be referred to as the 'geriatric giants' and are:

- mental confusion
- incontinence
- postural instability and falls
- immobility
- social breakdown.

It must be remembered that these are not diagnoses and are often the tip of a pathological iceberg, the bulk of which remains unseen and which will require careful diagnostic assessment to uncover. A diagrammatic example of this is seen in Figure 3.3 in which the presenting problem was falls but the underlying acute medical diagnosis was asthma.

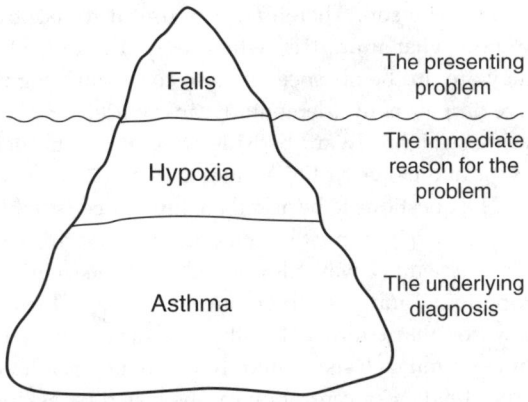

Fig. 3.3 The presenting problem is often the 'tip of the iceberg', with the underlying diagnosis not always apparent.

Thus it can be seen that any medical condition leading, for example, to hypoxia, could present with falls, confusion or incontinence or a combination of these. There are many permutations and it is part of the skill of geriatric medicine to unravel the clinical picture and gain an understanding of what is happening in any individual acutely ill elderly patient. History-taking is often difficult because of deafness, dysphasia, mental confusion or anxiety.

It is advisable, if possible, to corroborate the patient's history with information from a relative or friend. In such a case, first take as full a history as possible from the patient, and then while he or she is being prepared for physical examination, the relative's version of the history should also be obtained.

If there is any doubt as to the reliability of the patient's history because of either loss of memory or clouding of consciousness, then tests of memory and awareness should be built into the history-taking.

Often the patient's acute confusion is so severe as to be obvious, but in the more subtle cases it will be necessary to do a more formal assessment.

It is usually possible to do this by asking patients what they do all day and particularly whether they read, listen to the radio or watch the television, and if so what have they recently read, listened to or watched, and then see whether the answers make sense. When patients are acutely confused their sense of time tends to be the first thing to be impaired, then sense of place and finally sense of person. Therefore, it is useful to ask the subject what time it is, where they are and who they are. In the absence of acute confusion, cognitive impairment (dementia) can be detected by using straightforward bedside screening tests such as the abbreviated Mini Mental test score.

The questions to be asked are illustrated in Table 7.3 (see p. 57). It must be remembered that this test for dementia was developed in the United Kingdom and is therefore culturally biased towards that country. In other countries and cultures, similar tests would have to be modified accordingly. Concentration can be tested by asking the patient to perform the Serial Sevens test (100–7, 93–7, 86–7 etc.) or by reciting the months of the year forwards and then backwards.

The skillful clinician will introduce these tests quite naturally into the overall assessment of the patient, and it is possible to do this without causing offence.

Taking a systematic history from an elderly patient

Much of the history will be the same as in an adult patient of any age. Therefore, in this chapter we will emphasize those aspects of the history which are of particular importance in frail elderly subjects.

Special note should always be made of evidence of dysuric symptoms: for example, how many times the patient has to get up at night to pass urine, whether there is any incontinence and if so what is its nature. Always ask whether any falls have occurred in the previous year. If there have been any they must be described in detail.

It is often necessary to ask relatives whether there have been any episodes of mental confusion, abnormal behaviour, hallucinations etc.

Dizziness or lightheadedness is a symptom which most elderly people will confirm if asked directly. Therefore, as a symptom in its own right it tends to be of relatively little value.

However, if a distinct pattern of dizziness or lightheadedness can be uncovered this may aid the diagnosis considerably. For example, if it is associated with rotational vertigo it is likely to be due to vestibular disease, or if it only occurs on turning the neck it may be due to carotid sinus hypersensitivity or vertebral artery insufficiency. Faintness which only occurs when the patient stands is likely to be due to postural hypotension. There are many other examples and the clinician needs to use a knowledge of anatomy, physiology and pathology to get to the bottom of the symptom of dizziness in elderly people.

Always find out about diet, particularly if the patient lives alone. Sometimes this is best discovered by asking the patient to recall what has actually been eaten in the last 24 or 48 hours. It is important to know what social services are being provided, whether there is any family nearby and whether relatives are seen regularly.

It must be remembered that anxiety and depression are common in old age and are often difficult to detect. Therefore ask patients whether they are in good spirits, and always include in the history other questions which may help to assess the patients mental state: for example, do they enjoy their food?; do they sleep well?; are they prone to feelings of sadness or episodes of tearfulness? Try to get some idea about the patient's alcohol consumption. It is now known that alcohol abuse is not rare in elderly men and women and can often contribute to problems such as confusional states and falls.

The physical examination

The astute clinician will have been observing the patient, and therefore starting the physical examination, during the history-taking. Features such as the patient's posture, the presence of any tremors and the condition of the patient's skin are often noted well before the physical examination begins. As the patient approaches the couch for the examination a note must be made of the gait: does the patient walk safely?; is there any evidence of ataxia or any of the features of other neurological conditions such as Parkinson's disease?

Subtle degrees of ataxia will be brought to light by asking the patient to stand with the feet together, first with the eyes open and then closed. A normal person of any age will be able to stand still in this position, whereas those with a problem with balance or ataxia will lose balance quickly, particularly once the eyes are closed.

Much of the clinical examination will be along the same lines as in a person of any age and will not be considered in detail here. However, as with the history, there are a number of special factors which should be taken into consideration when examining an elderly patient. Some of these will be dealt with in other parts of this book. Nevertheless, a few general points in examination are explained in the rest of this chapter.

The weight should be measured and recorded for future reference. Since it is often not helpful to relate weight to the actual height of an old person, an estimate of height at maturity may be obtained by measuring the span of the outstretched arms from fingertip to fingertip. This will also give some idea of height loss due to age-related degenerative diseases of the spine and osteoporotic collapse of the vertebrae.

The skin becomes thinner through changes in collagen and may be so transparent over the backs of the hands that tendons and small veins are easily seen. Light trauma to such skin may produce haemorrhages called senile purpura.

These are distinguishable from ecchymosis by the fact that they only occur on the extensor surface of the hand and forearm and they do not change colour as they resolve. Clinically they are of little significance. Many patients with thin transparent skin will also have osteoporosis, particularly when both these conditions are the result of prolonged corticosteroid therapy. Senile keratosis, raised whitish yellow plaques of sodden-looking skin, is unsightly, but without clinical significance.

Muscle wasting increases with age and is easily seen in the face and hands. Loss of mass in the small muscles of the hands may exaggerate the size of the second and third metacarpo-phalangeal joints and is sometimes mistaken for rheumatoid arthritis. Particular attention should be paid to the breasts, the joints and feet, and the tongue and teeth.

Central nervous system

Power and coordination in the limbs may be rapidly estimated by having the patient perform three simple manoeuvres:

1. Stretch out the arms in front and see if the patient can maintain them in one position with the eyes closed. Drift of one of the arms from that position is an indicator of dyspraxia (or may be due to weakness) and should prompt a full examination for evidence of dyspraxia due to a cerebral hemisphere lesion.

2. The patient should tap the back of the hand quickly with the other hand and repeat this the other way around. This is an extremely useful screening test for ataxia.

3. The patient should perform the heel-knee test which is a very useful way of assessing ataxia, dyspraxia and pain on movement of the legs.

If abnormalities are found in any of these tests a very detailed examination should proceed.

It is often difficult to estimate muscle tone in elderly people because of guarding around osteoarthrotic joints. An unusual type of increase in muscle tone in old people is paratonic rigidity, sometimes known as gegenhalten, which is a manifestation of dyspraxia in patients with diffuse cerebral arteriosclerosis.

Deep tendon reflexes may be diminished by age-related change in the peripheral nerves, slowing conduction. In particular, ankle jerks are often difficult or impossible to elicit.

Sensation is usually retained, apart from vibration sense which again is often lost in the legs in older subjects and is not necessarily a sign of sensory neuropathy.

When examining the central nervous system always estimate the visual fields, looking especially for homonymous hemianopia in patients with stroke.

Primitive reflexes may emerge with ageing, particularly the palmomental and glabellar tap reflexes (see p. 31), or may be the result of age-associated disease such as stroke and multi-infarct dementia, which can lead to emergence of the snout, sucking, grasp and extensor plantar reflexes.

Cardiovascular system

On examining the cardiovascular system in old people it is particularly important to make a note of added heart sounds which may indicate the presence of incipient cardiac failure, and the murmurs of mitral incompetence and aortic stenosis which are common in old age and will require further assessment prior to treatment. This is discussed in Chapter 13.

Rhythm disorders are frequent and it is particularly important to detect the presence of atrial fibrillation. Blood pressure should be measured with the patient both lying and standing. The standing blood pressure should be measured after the patient has been resting in the lying position for at least 5 minutes, and then readings should be taken immediately after standing and at 2 minutes.

Auscultation over the carotid arteries for a bruit should always be performed and the presence or absence of peripheral pulses should be noted.

Respiratory system

It is notoriously difficult to assess the significance of basal lung crackles in old people. However, if the patient has crackles which persist after taking a few deep breaths they are more likely to be of clinical significance. Counting the respiratory rate is very helpful, and a rise in respiratory rate may be the first sign of respiratory infection or worsening cardiac failure. Elderly patients who use inhaler therapy should be asked to demonstrate their inhaler technique to make sure they are using the devices correctly.

The abdomen

Examination of the abdomen differs little in elderly people when compared to the young. However, it has already been mentioned that it is essential to check the state of the patient's mouth, particularly the teeth and tongue.

Within the abdomen the aorta of an old person is often easily felt and may be displaced if it is tortuous. An expansile aorta indicates the presence of an aortic aneurysm. The soundness of the abdominal wall may be judged by having the patient lift the head off the pillow. The presence of palpable faeces should always be noted.

Rectal examination should never be omitted because constipation is such a common complaint in old age, and an unsuspected carcinoma of the rectum is occasionally diagnosed by this means. It is sometimes difficult to distinguish between hard faecal masses in the rectum and a carcinoma and if there is any doubt, the examination should be repeated after emptying the rectum by an enema and by performing proctoscopy.

In patients with dysuric or vulvovaginal symptoms, the vulva should always be examined, and it is occasionally necessary to perform a bimanual examination of the vagina and pelvis.

Laboratory tests and special investigations

Of course, the choice of laboratory tests and other investigations will depend upon the clinical context and on the range of available equipment and expertise. Generally, the abnormalities found on biochemical and haematological testing have the same significance at any age. However, most of the published normal ranges for haematological and biochemical indices are based on two standard deviations about the mean for the local reference population. As physiological systems decline with age, the control of the chemical and cellular environment is often less accurate so that healthy elderly people quite often have test results which are slightly abnormal.

This must be borne in mind when interpreting the results of all tests, and is particularly important when batteries of screening tests are performed; a great deal of unnecessary time and money can be wasted by searching for the causes of marginally abnormal results in elderly patients when the overall clinical context has not been properly taken into account.

Furthermore, a number of age-related and degenerative diseases in old age cause biological and haematological changes which can make the interpretation of laboratory investigations more difficult than in young people. For example, asymptomatic Paget's disease will cause a rise in the blood alkaline phosphatase level and myelodysplasia often causes a persistent normochromic anaemia. Drug therapy in the elderly can also alter biochemical and haematological indices; for example, many old people taking a diuretic will have a slightly high blood urea.

However, there are some tests which have been shown to have a very high yield as screening tests in ill elderly people. These are listed in Box 3.1. Because anaemia, hypokalaemia and bone disease are so common in old age, a full blood count, a biochemical profile, and an estimate of serum electrolytes should always be done at the initial examination. Urinalysis for protein and sugar should always be carried out, and if dysuric symptoms are present a midstream specimen of urine should be sent for culture. It is good practice in hospital consultation to obtain an electrocardiogram (ECG) and chest radiograph at the first examination. Even if these reveal no treatable abnormality they may still be important as baseline information for the future. Special investigations will be discussed in context and these must always be undertaken if remediable pathology is suspected. It is often justifiable, and indeed important, to carry out tests to confirm the diagnosis, even if the illness is not thought to be treatable. In planning the patient's future an accurate prognosis is needed and sometimes, if these investigations are omitted because it is thought that the patient is too old, the wrong diagnosis will be made; this may seriously affect the management over a number of years. Since old people are so prone to constipation a special preparation is needed before sigmoidoscopy,

---

Box 3.1 Screening tests which give a high diagnostic yield in ill elderly patients in whom the diagnosis is not immediately clear

- Urine testing for glucose, blood and protein
- A full blood count
- Blood urea, creatinine, Na^+ and K^+
- Serum albumin, Ca^{++}, alkaline phosphatase and alanine aminotransferase (ALT)
- Blood sugar
- Chest radiograph
- Electrocardiogram
- Urine specimen for culture and microscopy

---

colonoscopy, barium enema and barium CT. Overnight admission to hospital is usually required in order to have a properly prepared patient and to save a lot of expensive professional time. Very often bowel preparation has to be carried out at home for several days beforehand in addition to this.

In disease of the central nervous system the limits of investigation are sometimes more difficult to define. There need be no hesitation in using noninvasive techniques such as computerized tomography or magnetic resonance imaging.

Similarly, as many old people are able to benefit from revascularization operations it may be perfectly appropriate for angiography of the cerebral, coronary or peripheral arteries to be performed.

In short, the full range of investigations should be available to elderly people but used judiciously to enable the clinician to make diagnoses and plan treatment which is likely to benefit the patient or enable an estimation to be made of prognosis.

Part 2

Major geriatric problems

4

Cerebral syndromes: brain disease in old age

Many of the most important problems in ill frail elderly people are at least partly due to brain disease. While many brain diseases are very similar in old age and in young adults there are certain conditions which are so overwhelmingly important in old age that they warrant a chapter of their own.

Arterial disease is a major cause of morbidity and disability in elderly patients in Europe, North America and some other industrialized societies. In the brain, arterial disease may cause one of a number of well-recognized syndromes in old people such as hemiplegia, but may also lead to less clear-cut clinical changes such as confusional states and poor balance. In addition, vascular changes may coexist with other pathological changes in the brain such as the senile plaques and neurofibrillary tangles of senile dementia, which are discussed in Chapter 20.

Furthermore, cerebral arterial insufficiency may predispose to an acute confusional disorder which is then precipitated by some further impairment of the function of cortical neurons whose blood supply is already critically diminished.

Thus superadded hypoxia due, for instance, to pneumonia or pulmonary oedema, hypotension in myocardial infarction, or toxaemia due to drugs or infection may cause a temporary derangement of a brain which is already made vulnerable by vascular insufficiency. These interactions are very important when considering the various cerebral syndromes in old people and help to account for their sometimes bewildering variety.

Cerebral circulation

The circulation of blood to the brain is supplied by the two internal carotid arteries and two vertebral arteries. The basic anatomy of this is shown in Figure 4.1. The student requires a reasonable knowledge of the blood supply to the brain in order to make sense of the various brain syndromes that occur when the normal supply is interrupted.

The common carotid arteries arise from the innominate artery on the right and directly from the aorta on the left. They divide into the internal and external carotids and there is some anastomosis between these two through the ophthalmic artery. On each side the internal carotid finally passes through the carotid canal to enter the skull and then divides into the anterior and middle cerebral arteries.

The vertebral arteries arise from the subclavian artery and pass backwards to enter the foramina of the upper six cervical vertebrae. The position of

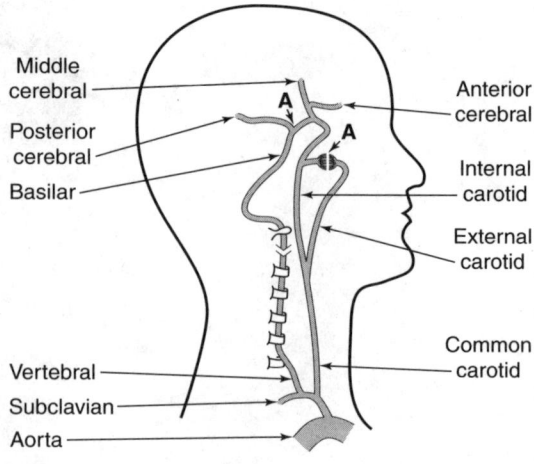

Fig. 4.1 Cerebral circulation. A = anastomosis.

these arteries is illustrated in Figures 4.2 and 4.3, from which it will be apparent that the vertebral arteries are susceptible to the effects of a number of pathological and ageing processes affecting the neck.

After passing through the transverse process of the atlas the vertebral arteries enter the skull from the foramen magnum. They lie on the dorsal part of the hind brain, coming together to form the basilar artery overlying the pons; after giving off the posterior inferior cerebellar arteries, the basilar artery divides into the two posterior cerebral arteries.

The most important anastomotic structure which ensures blood supply to the highly vulnerable cells of the brain, even if one of the four principal arteries is occluded, is the Circle of Willis, which is formed from the vessels already mentioned by an anterior communicating artery, joining the two anterior cerebral arteries and, by two posterior communicating arteries, joining the middle and posterior cerebral arteries.

All the structures of the cerebral circulation become particularly vulnerable in old age.

The carotid circulation in the neck is an important site for the formation of atheromatous plaques which occur particularly at sites of bifurcation and are especially common in the internal carotid artery at its origin. The Circle of Willis also may be functionally impaired by extensive formation of atheromatous plaques. In addition, all the smaller arteries to the brain may be affected by arteriosclerotic change including atheromatous plaques, medial fibrosis, hyalinization and calcification.

An important change which sometimes affects vertebrobasilar circulation is degeneration of the intervertebral discs in the cervical spine caused by age-related loss of water, fibrosis and changes in the mucopolysaccharide composition of the nucleus pulposus. This results in the intervertebral discs becoming squashed with narrowing of the disc space and bulging of the disc margin so that the intervertebral ligaments and their attached periosteum are pushed away from the vertebral bodies. This results in new bone formation with the development of osteophytes, and this leads to the condition which is generally known as cervical spondylosis. The intervertebral discs account for about 25% of the length of the spine and so disc degeneration is one of the reasons for loss of height with ageing.

The clinical significance of cervical spondylosis is not certain. Such changes are almost universal in very old people, only a few of whom develop cerebral syndromes which could conceivably be due to interruption of flow in the vertebrobasilar arterial system. Nevertheless, some individuals do develop

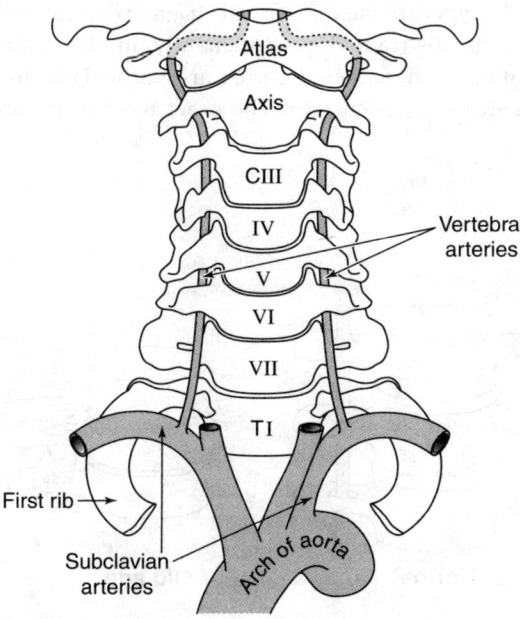

Fig. 4.2 The vertebral arteries.

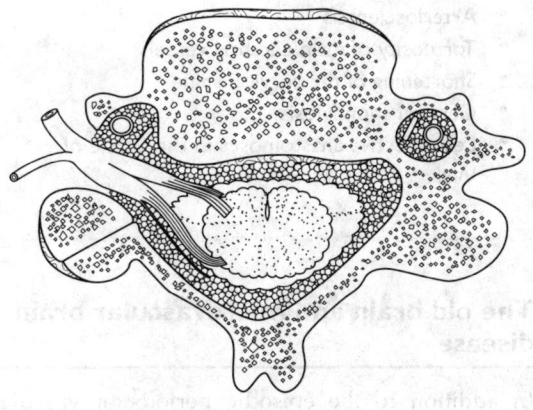

Fig. 4.3 Cross-section of a cervical vertebral showing the vertebral arteries within the vertebral canals.

symptoms which are related to neck movements and these patients probably do have a genuine causal relationship between their cervical spondylosis and their symptoms.

In such people it is likely that osteophytes which are formed around the margin of the vertebral body impinge on the vertebral arteries and in certain positions of the neck may partially occlude them. Also, secondary loss of height in the cervical spine, combined with degenerative changes in the arteries themselves, may lead to tortuosity of the vertebral arteries and thereby make them vulnerable to kinking and occlusion in certain neck positions. Figures 4.4 and 4.5 demonstrate these changes diagrammatically.

It is important to stress, however, that elderly patients with symptoms such as lightheadedness, dizziness or syncope should not have these clinical presentations explained away merely because of the demonstration of cervical spondylosis on a radiograph of the cervical spine. Many other conditions can cause similar symptoms and a proper diagnostic work-up is necessary.

The key factors which render the cerebral circulation vulnerable in elderly people are listed in Box 4.1.

> ## Box 4.1 Factors making the cerebral circulation of old people vulnerable
>
> - Atheromatous plaques
> - Arteriosclerosis
> - Tortuosity of main cerebral vessels
> - Shortening of the cervical spine
> - Cervical spondylosis
> - Less effective anastomoses in the Circle of Willis

The old brain and microvascular brain disease

In addition to the episodic periods of vascular insufficiency referred to above, prolonged widespread impairment of cerebral circulation leads

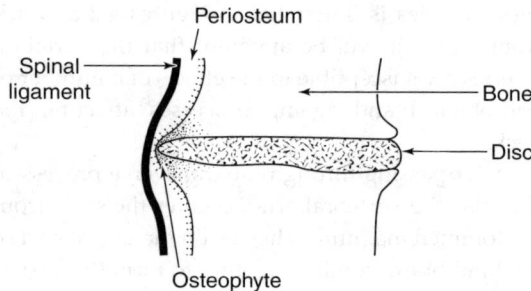

Fig. 4.4 Disc degeneration.

eventually to cerebral atrophy and a number of other characteristic pathological changes. These are thought to be due to degenerative changes in very small arteries and arterioles, and they lead to the presence of small smooth-walled cavities containing minute tortuous arteries, which are particularly in evidence in the basal ganglia and in the central white matter of the brain. These are sometimes referred to as 'état criblé' and 'état lacunaire'. Microaneurysm formation also occurs, particularly in subjects who are hypertensive or diabetic. All of these changes become increasingly common with advancing age and there is evidence that they are accelerated in subjects with hypertension, diabetes and hyperlipidaemia. Small haemorrhages and infarcts distributed predominantly in the white matter of the cerebral cortex are particularly frequent in hypertensives. The exact mechanism for

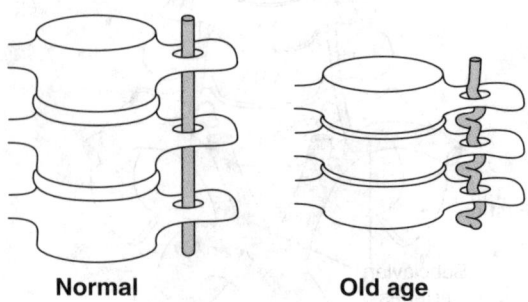

Fig. 4.5 Changes in cervical spine as a result of disc degeneration.

this is uncertain but it seems likely that both microembolism and obstructive microangiopathy play a role in the pathogenesis.

Conditions affecting the whole brain: cerebral arteriosclerosis and multi-infarct dementia

In patients with generalized cerebral arteriosclerosis and multiple small infarcts throughout the brain a characteristic clinical picture emerges, the main features of which are as follows:

- generalized apraxia
- generalized hypertonia with brisk tendon reflexes
- a tendency to lean backwards
- a characteristic disorder of gait
- dementia
- incontinence of the uninhibited neurogenic bladder type.

The patient displays paratonic rigidity, sometimes also referred to as gegenhalten, a form of hypertonia in which the patient seems unable to relax the muscles when the limbs are being held by another person. This is sometimes referred to as being quasivolitional because the impression that the examiner gets is that the patient is positively resisting attempts to move the limbs passively.

The rigidity is inconstant in that it does not occur in the same position of the limb every time; nor does it interfere with the range of active movement through which the patient can put the limb when it is not being held by someone else.

It thus appears that this rigidity is an inability to relate to movements when in contact with another person and is therefore a form of apraxia. Similarly, when nursing staff roll such patients towards them when they are handling them on a bed, the patients immediately show widespread muscular rigidity, often clinging to the nurse's clothes.

Another form of this apraxia is seen when someone tries to assist such a patient to rise and walk. The patient will seem to lean backwards and again go into a state of generalized hypertonia, though if asked to get up and walk without being in contact with another person the same patient may be able to do so without great difficulty.

The typical gait disturbance seen in cerebral arterial disease with multiple infarcts is described as the Petren gait or astasia abasia.

This is characterized by shuffling and a tendency for the feet to seem intermittently glued to the floor. The feet are often pushed into the ground. However, if the patient is asked to step over a stick held at a height of about 30 cm (12 inches), this can often be achieved without difficulty. This gait is distinct from the festinating gait of Parkinson's disease which is described in greater detail later in this chapter.

The tendon reflexes are usually very brisk and in the early stages of the condition the plantar responses remain flexor, though in the late stages they often become extensor.

The findings described above are the most important ones in the clinical assessment of a patient with cerebral arteriosclerosis. However, a number of primitive reflexes often emerge in this condition and if present they indicate widespread generalized cerebral impairment. These include:

1. *The grasp reflex.* A stimulus of moving touch, or touch and pressure, over the radial side of the hand in the direction of the fingers leads to a brief contraction of the flexor muscles of the hands and fingers.

If the stimulus then moves to the flexing fingers, pulling against them, there is a rapid increase in the strength of the contraction. The reflex becomes more sensitive if repeated two or three times, a phenomenon known as temporal summation.

2. *Forced groping.* If the palm is touched when the patient has closed eyes, the fingers close and the hand moves in the direction that the stimulus appears to come from.

3. *Snout reflex.* Tapping on the upper lip leads to pouting of the lips.

4. *Sucking reflex.* An object such as a pencil in contact with the lips produces the muscle contractions appropriate to sucking.

5. *Palmomental reflex.* A nonpainful stimulus such as a scratch from an orange stick applied to the hypothenar eminence produces a contraction of the mentalis muscle.

6. *Glabellar tap reflex.* The glabella, the midpoint between the orbital ridges, is tapped

rhythmically with the finger. The normal person will blink synchronously with the tapping for a few moments and then stop. The sign is positive when the subject continues to blink synchronously or the eyelids go into spasm.

The last two, the palmomental and glabellar reflexes, may be positive in up to 50% of people over the age of 75 and are therefore of less clinical significance than the others mentioned.

Other important neurological features of multi-infarct brain disease include perseveration of speech, urinary incontinence of the uninhibited neurogenic bladder type, dysarthria, pseudobulbar palsy and loss of upward gaze.

Transient ischaemic attacks

A transient ischaemic attack (TIA) is an episode of focal loss of brain function lasting for a few minutes or hours from which full recovery occurs within 24 hours.

When the symptoms and signs last for more than 24 hours but less than 72 hours, the term 'reversible ischaemic neurological deficit' (RIND) is used. The pathology of RINDs is more or less the same as that of TIAs.

TIAs rarely cause loss of consciousness. The symptoms and signs vary depending on which part of the brain is affected and TIAs may occur either in the carotid territory or the vertebrobasilar territory. Although a full understanding of the pathogenesis of TIAs has not yet been achieved, it is thought that the majority are due to embolization of small platelet aggregates arising on the surface of atheromatous plaques in the larger vessels of the carotid and vertebrobasilar arterial systems.

An enormous variety of symptoms can be caused by TIAs but the most common include transient monoparesis or hemiparesis; transient hemiparaesthesiae or a hemianaesthesia; speech disorders including dysphasia when the dominant hemisphere is involved; and dysarthria is a common feature of vertebrobasilar TIAs. Monocular loss of vision (amaurosis fugax) occurs when microemboli temporarily block the retinal artery on one side. Because the microemboli are usually arising from the same diseased artery, the symptoms of

TIAs tend to be the same during each attack in any given individual.

TIAs in the vertebrobasilar system are an important cause of collapse, though the differential diagnosis is usually not difficult as there are often other brain stem physical signs present if the patient is examined before full recovery occurs.

The prognostic significance of TIAs

TIAs in the carotid territory will lead to a stroke in about 30% of patients over a 3-year period if no treatment is given. Vertebrobasilar TIAs appear to confer less of a risk, though some patients do develop a full-blown posterior circulation stroke.

The presence of TIAs is often an indication of more widespread arterial disease and a substantial number of people with TIAs will develop significant ischaemic heart disease including myocardial infarction in the succeeding years.

Treatment

Large-scale trials over the last 10 years have provided clinicians with a considerable amount of guidance in the management and treatment of patients with TIAs. One approach, based on the current evidence, is outlined in Figure 4.6.

It can be seen that the mainstay of treatment is with aspirin, which through its effect on prostaglandin synthetase, reduces platelet aggregation. Treatment with aspirin will significantly reduce the frequency of TIAs and reduce the risk of a full-blown stroke in the carotid territory. The benefits of aspirin in vertebrobasilar TIAs are less clear-cut but there is evidence of benefit.

Recent research has shown that carotid endarterectomy in addition to aspirin will only produce net benefit in patients with severe stenosis in which there is a greater than 70% reduction in carotid artery diameter measured by Doppler ultrasound. All patients found to have carotid stenosis should be investigated for ischaemic heart disease. Also, of course, treatment of TIAs with aspirin will have a secondary benefit in those who do have ischaemic heart disease.

Some patients who continue to have frequent TIAs when taking aspirin can benefit from anticoagulation with warfarin, providing there are no

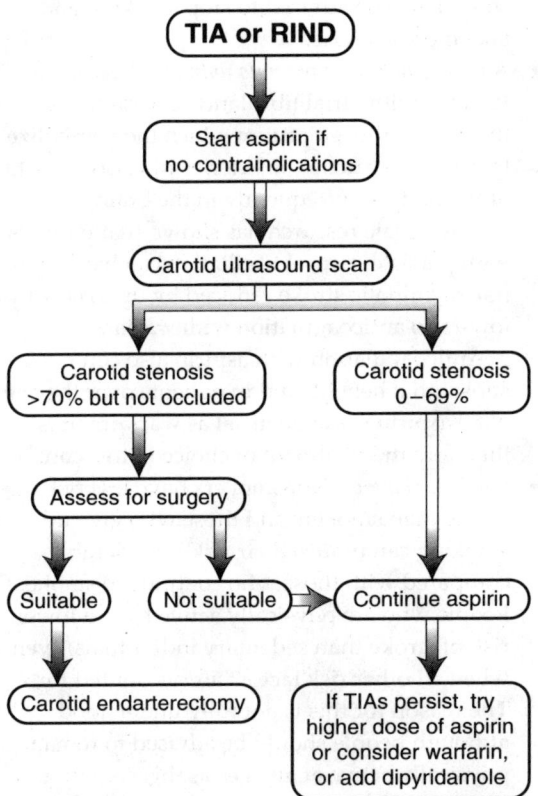

Fig. 4.6 Scheme for treating transient ischaemic attacks (TIAs) and reversible ischaemic neurological deficits (RINDSs).

contraindications such as uncontrolled hypertension, peptic ulceration or a tendency to fall. Adding dipyridamole is also effective.

Stroke

Stroke is an important disease in old age, partly because the incidence rises with age and becomes particularly common in people over the age of 75, and partly because it often leads to considerable degrees of neurological impairment and therefore functional problems and dependency.

Definition of stroke

Stroke can be defined as a sudden loss of neurological function from a vascular cause.

Haemorrhages on to the surface of the brain,

such as subarachnoid, subdural and extradural haemorrhages, are not usually included in this definition. Therefore, stroke is usually the result of interruption of blood flow to a part of the brain as a result of thrombosis, embolism, or haemorrhage into the brain substance. Box 4.2 summarizes the main underlying pathology leading to these causes of stroke although the list is by no means exhaustive.

Box 4.2 Causes of stroke

- Cerebral thrombosis
- Atherosclerosis
- Thrombogenic states
- Hyperviscosity
- Severe dehydration

Cerebral thrombosis
- Thromboembolism from atheromatous plaques in the arterial system to the brain
- Thrombi arising in the left ventricle, particularly after myocardial infarction
- Thrombi arising in the left atrium, particularly in atrial fibrillation
- Bacterial endocarditis

Cerebral haemorrhage
- Rupture of microaneurysms (especially diabetics and hypertensives)
- haemorrhagic transformation of a cerebral infarction

Whether the stroke is caused by infarction or haemorrhage, the clinical picture will depend on the extent of neurological damage in the brain substance. Strokes sometimes worsen in the first couple of days after the onset as a result of cerebral oedema around the infarct or haemorrhage, extension of the stroke by further thrombosis or by bleeding from vessels within a cerebral infarct with consequent expansion of the damaged area.

Risk factors for stroke

These are summarized in Box 4.3. It can be seen that

some risk factors are not modifiable, some can be managed and altered to a certain extent, while others can be avoided altogether.

This is a very important issue because a great deal of physical morbidity and mortality in older people could be avoided if some of the risk factors could be controlled more rigorously, and listed below are some of the most useful and rewarding approaches to the reduction of stroke risk.

Box 4.3 Risk factors for stroke

Unavoidable risks
- Age
- Strong family history of stroke disease

Partially modifiable risk factors
- Hypertension
- Diabetes mellitus
- Atrial fibrillation
- Myocardial infarction
- Hyperlipidemia
- Sedentary lifestyle

Avoidable risk factors
- Tobacco smoking
- In young people abuse of drugs which can cause very high blood pressure (BP), such as amphetamines and ecstasy

---

Recent research has shown that some of these risk factors can be substantially modified and lead to significant reduction in the risk of stroke. These include:

- *Treatment of hypertension.* Research has shown that treating hypertension will reduce the risk of stroke in patients of all ages. People with a systolic blood pressure (BP) persistently above 160 mmHg or diastolic BP above 95 mmHg should receive treatment. Furthermore, other studies have shown that in older people with isolated systolic hypertension, treatment causes a fall in the stroke incidence. Of course, it is necessary to control all other risk factors in order to get the best benefits, so such patients

should also be advised to stop smoking and take more exercise.

- *Anticoagulation in patients with atrial fibrillation.* Patients with atrial fibrillation can develop thrombi in the left atrium which then embolize to cause obstruction to arteries in various parts of the body, but frequently in the brain.

  Large-scale research has shown that patients with persistent atrial fibrillation can have their risk of embolic stroke reduced by up to 60% by low-ratio anticoagulation with warfarin.

  Anticoagulation with aspirin also confers a substantial benefit, and in patients over the age of 80 aspirin is as beneficial as warfarin; it is therefore the treatment of choice in this context.

- *Lifestyle changes.* Nonsmokers have less risk of stroke than smokers and those who give up smoking can reduce their risk considerably compared with those who continue to smoke. People who are physically active have a lower risk of stroke than sedentary individuals, even when all other risk factors are accounted for. The reason for this is not fully understood although people should be advised to remain physically active at all ages as this confers a range of physical and psychological benefits in addition to the reduction of stroke risk.

The classification of stroke

Of course, the clinical picture of stroke varies enormously and depends entirely on which part of the brain has been damaged. Some classifications are very complex and the student can find these in large specialist textbooks.

However, a useful classification, which enables us to understand the extent of damage caused by stroke and also gives some useful insights into prognosis, is outlined below; it uses clinical information to determine which broad arterial territory the stroke has occurred in. This clinical classification correlates well with the result of a computerized tomography (CT) head scan.

Classification of stroke by arterial territory. The classification outlined in Box 4.4 was first proposed by Bamford in the early 1990s. It applies to cerebral infarction rather than haemorrhage, though it must be remembered that only about 10%

of strokes are due to cerebral haemorrhage and so the classification is useful for the majority of patients with stroke.

Although the clinician must always take individual variation into account when assessing the functional loss from stroke and trying to predict the prognosis, this classification has proved to be broadly helpful in this respect.

Box 4.4 Clinical classification of stroke due to infarction

1. **Lacunar infarction (LACI)**
   - Caused by obstruction of a deep perforating artery leading to a small deep infarct
   - Clinical presentation as *one* of the following:
   — pure motor stroke
   — pure sensory stroke
   — ataxic hemiparesis
   — sensorimotor stroke
   - Without a visual field defect or new disturbance of higher cortical function

2. **Total anterior circulation infarction (TACI)**
   - Caused by occlusion of the main trunk of the middle cerebral artery
   - Clinical presentation is with *all* of the following:
   — hemiplegia
   — hemianopia
   — new disturbance of higher cerebral function, e.g. dysphasia or dyspraxia

3. **Partial anterior circulation infarction (PACI)**
   - Caused by obstruction of a branch of the middle cerebral artery
   - Clinical features can include *any* of the following combinations:
   — motor/sensory deficit and hemianopia
   — motor/sensory deficit and new higher cerebral dysfunction
   — new higher cerebral dysfunction and hemianopia

Box 4.4 Clinical classification of stroke due to infarction (contd)

   — pure motor/sensory deficit less extensive than for LACI (e.g. monoparesis)
   — new higher cerebral dysfunction alone
   — combinations of the above, but within the same hemisphere

4. **Posterior circulation infarction (POCI)**
   - Caused by occlusion of a vessel in the vertebrobasilar system
   - Patients can present with *any* of the following:
   — ipsilateral cranial nerve palsy and contralateral motor and/or sensory deficit
   — bilateral motor and/or sensory deficit
   — disordered conjugate eye movement
   — cerebellar dysfunction without long tract deficit
   — isolated hemianopia or cortical blindness
   — any of the above, plus new disturbance of higher cortical function

---

Differential diagnosis of stroke

In the differential diagnosis of stroke it is important to exclude subdural haematoma, particularly in patients whose level of consciousness fluctuates over a number of days and who also demonstrate a hemiparesis. Subdural haematoma is often related to a history of trauma to the head but this is present quite often in patients with cerebral infarct or haemorrhage because they fall. The other important diagnostic classification is a subarachnoid haemorrhage which again may produce hemiparesis, though more often the neurological loss is more diffuse.

Typically, there is intense generalized headache, often worse in the occiput with neck stiffness and photophobia. It must be noted that headache is a fairly frequent symptom in haemorrhagic stroke, particularly if blood leaks to the surface of the brain and enters the subarachnoid space.

Investigation of stroke

CT scanning is available in the general hospitals of most developed countries, and when this is available the majority of patients with stroke should have a scan. This quickly enables the clinician to differentiate cerebral infarction from cerebral haemorrhage and also helps to rule out the important differential diagnoses of subdural haematoma and subarachnoid haemorrhage. It would also help to diagnose the more unusual causes of stroke such as bleeding into a tumour and haemorrhagic transformation of a cerebral infarction. Magnetic resonance imaging (MRI) scanning is also widely available and gives much the same information in patients with stroke.

Treatment of stroke

This is a large and rapidly changing field of medicine and it is likely that we will see major advances over the next 10 years.

At the time of writing, the role of various treatments for acute stroke is not entirely clear. Trials of thrombolysis in very early stroke have been carried out though no definite benefit was demonstrated. New neuroprotective agents are under investigation and may well prove to be of value once their exact role has been properly defined. Anticoagulation with heparin does not appear to confer definite benefit in strokes generally, though there is evidence that early treatment with aspirin helps to reduce the incidence of early recurrence of stroke in patients with cerebral infarction.

Primary prevention of stroke

This is probably one of the major aspects of stroke treatment, and the most important approaches to primary prevention, based on large-scale trials, are listed below:

- anticoagulation in patients with chronic atrial fibrillation (see p. 34)
- aspirin therapy in patients with transient ischaemic attacks
- treatment of hypertension
- stopping smoking
- physically active lifestyle.

There are probably also benefits from the control of hyperlipidemia, good control of diabetes, weight reduction and a diet which is not too rich in saturated fat, though these benefits are less clear-cut than those listed above.

Secondary prevention of stroke

Patients who have already had a stroke can have the risk of a further stroke reduced by certain measures. These are listed below:

- by applying the primary prevention measures listed above
- low-dose aspirin therapy in patients with cerebral infarction.

The longer-term management of a patient with stroke

If a patient survives the acute phase of a stroke there is frequently a considerable amount of residual neurological impairment. This usually has a tremendous physical and emotional impact on the patient, relatives and friends, and the patient will require a carefully thought-out programme of rehabilitation to reduce the consequences of that impairment to a minimum, leaving the patient with as little handicap as possible.

In Chapter 21 later in this book the process of rehabilitation is described in more detail.

Vertebrobasilar syndromes

The vertebral and basilar arteries supply blood to the hind brain, the cerebellum and occipital cortices. Ischaemia in these areas may produce impairment of neuroregulatory functions.

These include, particularly, reflex posture, the maintenance of blood pressure, and of temperature regulation and the vomiting centre. Vertebrobasilar artery insufficiency therefore may be associated with falling, ataxia, nystagmus, giddiness, nausea and vomiting, episodes of hypotension and impairment of thermoregulation. Involvement of both occipital cortices may produce cortical blindness, and if only one is involved the patient may have homonomous hemianopia with macular sparing or visual hallucinations. Involvement of the cranial nerve nuclei may produce dysphagia, dysarthria, ophthalmoplegia, facial hemiparesis, hemianesthesia, peri-oral paraesthesia and vertigo.

Strokes occurring in the posterior circulation territory (POCI strokes) have been referred to above, as have vertebrobasilar transient ischaemic attacks. However, another important vertebrobasilar syndrome is that of drop attacks, and this phenomenon is described below.

Drop attacks

Drop attacks constitute a controversial area of medicine with an uncertain aetiology and a fairly broad differential diagnosis. Nevertheless, many clinicians hold the view that arterial insufficiency in the vertebrobasilar territory is at least one of the causes of drop attacks. In a typical drop attack the patient falls without warning or loss of consciousness and is often unable to rise immediately from the floor. Some patients describe momentary dizziness or vertigo before they fall and some are able to pick themselves up straight away. Typically, the patient who falls as a result of a drop attack crumples to the ground and consequently injuries are less common than in those who crash to the ground unconscious.

One theory is that drop attacks are due to sudden occlusion of both vertebral arteries as a result of kinking or impingement by cervical vertebral osteophytes when the patient moves the neck. Sudden loss of blood to the hind brain and cerebellum leads to a sudden loss of the reflex mechanisms for the maintenance of posture and so the patient falls.

It is suggested that the inability to rise immediately from the ground in some patients is because reflex posture does not return until there is sensory input into the proprioceptive system, which requires pressure on the soles of the feet and transmission of weight through the lower limbs. Certainly, once the patient who has had a drop attack is assisted into the standing position, walking can usually continue immediately.

The differential diagnosis of drop attacks is included in Box 4.5.

> ### Box 4.5 Differential diagnosis of drop attacks
>
> - A drop attack due to true vertebrobasilar insufficiency
> - Carotid sinus hypersensitivity with sudden severe bradycardia and/or hypotension
> - Vertebrobasilar transient ischaemic attack
> - Postural hypotension (usually a consistent relationship to posture and preceding faintness)

It must be noted that for patients who describe definite loss of consciousness a diagnosis of a drop attack should not be made. Such patients are more likely to have severe postural hypotension, a cardiac arrhythmia or epilepsy.

The treatment of drop attacks

In patients with frequent drop attacks, general measures to minimize injury are the most important aspect of treatment. These are as follows:

- The patient should be accompanied when performing hazardous tasks such as climbing the stairs.
- Fires and other hazardous appliances should be guarded.
- The patient and carers should be given an explanation of the drop attack and instructions by the physiotherapist on how to get the patient into the upright position again.

Investigations should be carried out to rule out the important differential diagnoses, particularly cardiac arrhythmias, postural hypotension and carotid sinus hypersensitivity, as these may respond to specific treatments. In a patient in whom neck movement is clearly related to symptoms (a relatively small proportion of the total) and where carotid sinus hypersensitivity has been ruled out, it is worth trying a cervical collar to limit neck movements. This should be reasonably close-fitting and comfortable. The collar does not need to be worn in bed at night but should be put on before getting out of bed in the morning. If the cervical collar does not alter the patient's symptoms it should be abandoned.

Our knowledge of the causes and management of drop attacks is as yet incomplete. Although compression of vessels by neck movement is a good theory it has yet to be proved and it is very unusual to be able to reproduce a drop attack by getting a patient to move the neck in different directions during examination in clinic or in a hospital ward.

Great care must be exercised before attributing dizziness and falls in old people to cervical spondylosis. A very large proportion of elderly people will have spondylitic change in their cervical spine radiologically and this will be of clinical importance in only a small proportion. On the other hand, cervical osteophytes may impinge on cervical nerve roots causing muscle wasting and tingling in the hands or occipital headache. Also, the osteophytes can compress the spinal cord to produce varying degrees of paraparesis or even tetraparesis.

Parkinson's disease

Parkinsonism is common in old age and our understanding of the neurology and neurochemistry of this condition has advanced greatly in recent years. Idiopathic Parkinson's disease is progressive, and although drug treatment is of great help in ameliorating the disease the patients become increasingly impaired and often require considerable support from their carers, health services and social services.

For a detailed account of the pathology and neurology of this condition the student is referred to major neurological textbooks. However, outlined below are some important features of idiopathic Parkinson's disease and related conditions.

Classical idiopathic Parkinson's disease

This is the typical paralysis agitans which often begins in late middle age but may have its onset in old age. In the early stages the patient may simply note a typical pill-rolling resting tremor in one upper limb. At this stage the disease is not disabling, though it often provokes a great deal of anxiety. Later, the fully developed picture is one of severe bradykinesia with difficulty initiating move-

ment, tremor, rigidity, excessive salivation, paucity of facial expression, autonomic disorders and mild cognitive impairment.

Arterio-sclerotic Parkinsonism

This term is often used to describe the extra-pyramidal features which often accompany multi-infarct brain disease. The features of cerebral arteriosclerosis, such as generalized hypertonia and the emergence of primitive reflexes, tend to be present and are accompanied by a number of features seen in classical Parkinson's disease such as bradykinesia and sometimes tremor. It is assumed that the condition is due to vascular damage in the mid-brain, and there is some evidence from modern imaging techniques that this is the case. There tends not to be any response to treatment with L-dopa.

Drug-induced Parkinsonism

This is common in old people and is usually associated with treatment with phenothiazine tranquillizers, and occasionally with tricyclic antidepressants. It is usually, but not always, reversible when the drug is withdrawn. When the drug needs to be continued, side-effects can be controlled with anticholinergic agents such as benzhexol.

Other causes of Parkinsonism

These are numerous but mostly rare. Perhaps the best-known example is multisystem atrophy (the Shy Drager syndrome), where progressive dysfunction in the extra-pyramidal system is associated with atrophy and dysfunction in other neurological systems, particularly the autonomic nervous system and upper motor neurons.

Differential diagnosis of a Parkinsonian tremor

The tremor in idiopathic Parkinson's disease is a coarse tremor which occurs with the limbs at rest while the patient is awake. It tends to be abolished by movement and is absent during sleep. When the hands are involved the fingers move in a typical pill-rolling fashion. This enables it to be distinguished from the tremor of cerebellar dysfunction, which is typically ataxic and is exaggerated by movement; and from senile tremor, which is more generalized, more rapid, tends to be worsened by movement and is not associated with the other features of Parkinson's disease.

Movement disorders associated with other forms of damage to the basal ganglia, such as athetosis, chorea or hemiballismus, are so clearly different from a Parkinsonian tremor that the differential diagnosis is not usually a problem.

Treatment of Parkinson's disease

Idiopathic Parkinson's disease is associated with severe depletion of dopamine in the substantia nigra of the basal ganglia. The mainstay of treatment is to enhance the availability of dopamine by treatment with L-dopa in combination with a dopa-decarboxylase inhibitor to diminish the peripheral breakdown of L-dopa to dopamine outside the central nervous system, and thereby allow high concentrations of L-dopa and therefore dopamine within the central nervous system. Lower doses of L-dopa may thus be used, which leads to fewer side-effects. The main side-effects of L-dopa are those arising within the central nervous system, particularly dyskinesia. Figure 4.7 illustrates the point at which the various drugs available for the treatment of Parkinson's disease act on dopaminergic transmission in the basal ganglia.

The use of many of these agents is a specialist field and therefore outside the scope of this book, though in general it should be emphasized that L-dopa therapy forms a first-line treatment, with selegiline and pergolide being the most important adjunctive treatments. Most of the other drugs are used only in special circumstances.

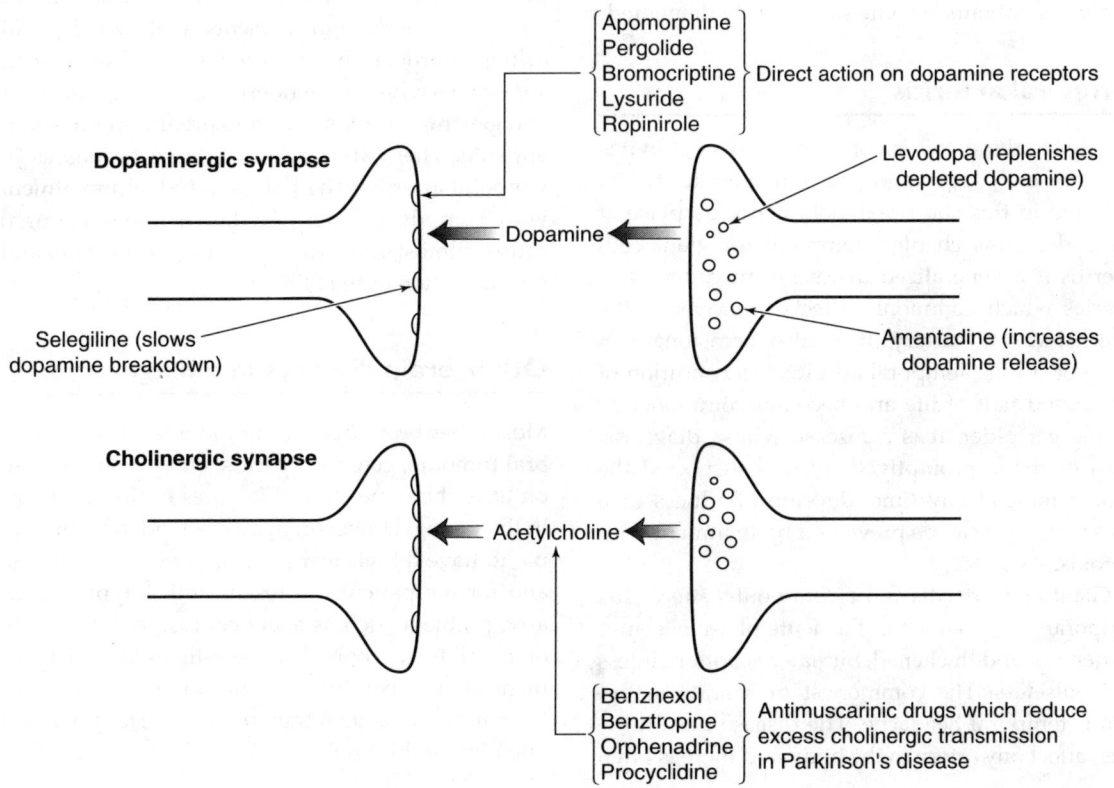

Fig. 4.7 The site of action of various drugs used in Parkinson's disease.

Longer-term management of Parkinson's disease

Though drug therapy is very helpful, it is rarely sufficient on its own, particularly when the patient with Parkinson's disease has progressed to the point where drugs are only having a minimal effect. At this stage the patient often requires considerable help from physiotherapists and occupational therapists, and the full range of facilities available from a rehabilitation team. The disease is distressing, and psychological and social support from rehabilitation staff in day hospitals, day centres and organizations such as the Parkinson's Disease Society becomes at least as important as drug therapy.

Patients with Parkinson's disease often become depressed, and the diagnosis is frequently overlooked because the patient may have lost normal facial expression. The evidence is that response to antidepressant treatment is quite good under these circumstances. Cognitive impairment is also a feature of idiopathic Parkinson's disease, and a proportion of patients become significantly demented.

Temporal arteritis

Strictly speaking, this is not a brain disease, but it is of sufficient importance in old people to be included in this short textbook; hence its place at the end of this chapter. Temporal (or giant cell) arteritis is a generalized disease of medium-sized arteries which commonly affects branches of the external carotid artery. It is also occasionally a cause of stroke. Temporal arteritis is a condition of the second half of life and becomes commoner as people get older. It is a disease whose diagnosis must be made promptly, for if it is suspected the patient may, at any time, develop blindness or a stroke and this can be prevented by treatment with steroids.

Giant cell arteritis most commonly affects the temporal artery, which in the acute phase becomes tender, hot and thickened, but later is both painless and pulseless. The commonest presenting symptom is temporal headache. The disease may, however, affect any artery in the body and there is often constitutional disturbance such as malaise, fatigue, generalized aches and pains, a reduced appetite or low-grade fever. The retinal artery is the second most commonly affected and this may be bilateral, leading to impairment or total loss of vision.

The diagnosis of giant cell arteritis may be suspected by elevation of the erythrocyte sedimentation rate (ESR) and confirmed by a biopsy of the affected artery. These investigations should not be awaited, however, before treatment is started. Blood should be removed for ESR measurement and the patient started on 40–60 mg prednisolone per day. This can usually be reduced to a dose of 10–20 mg within 2 weeks and a maintenance dose of around 5–10 mg per day for the next year. It is then sometimes possible to withdraw steroid therapy, though the disease may reactivate and require further treatment. People sometimes require treatment indefinitely.

Another disease which is closely associated with giant cell arteritis and also common in the elderly is polymyalgia rheumatica. This is a disease of joints and not muscle and presents with widespread aching, particularly around the shoulder girdle, sometimes with mild tenderness, a low-grade fever and general symptoms such as tiredness and a poor appetite. There are no focal arterial lesions as in temporal arteritis. The ESR is raised and treatment with steroids (15 mg per day is often enough) causes almost immediate relief of symptoms and normalization of the ESR.

Other brain diseases in old age

Most other brain diseases in old age, such as cerebral tumours, cerebral abscess, encephalitis and so on have the same clinical features in the elderly as in the young. However, there is a tendency for people to have a less clear-cut presentation in old age and for the patient to present with a typical geriatric problem such as acute confusion, immobility or inability to cope. The investigation and treatment of such conditions is no different in old age from in the young so they do not warrant detailed attention in this book.

Disorders of the autonomic nervous system

Introduction

Impairment of the autonomic nervous system becomes increasingly common with age, though frank autonomic failure remains relatively rare. Nevertheless, a number of common and important clinical syndromes are due, at least in part, to reduced efficiency of the autonomic nervous system in older people. These include accidental hypothermia, postural hypotension, some forms of bladder dysfunction, swallowing difficulties and disordered motility of the large bowel. To a certain extent these changes are the effect of ageing itself on the autonomic nervous system, though in some people the dysfunction arises as the result of pathological processes such as diabetes mellitus. The final clinical effect is often multifactorial and occurs as a result of dysfunction in the autonomic nerves themselves, underperformance of the hypothalamic autonomic controller and impairment to various effector organs such as vascular smooth muscle and myocardium. Furthermore, drugs and environmental factors may contribute, as may the patient's general morbidity and metabolic status. Therefore, it is very important to look at the patient as a whole when assessing dysfunction in the autonomic nervous system.

Age-related changes in the autonomic nervous system

Research in recent years has given us some understanding of how the autonomic nervous system changes in old age. Certainly there is a reduced response to sympathetic nerve stimulation or the infusion of catecholamines, and there is an age-related decrease in beta 1 and beta 2 adrenoreceptor sensitivity. The observation that many old people have higher baseline levels of plasma noradrenaline than young people may in part be a compensatory mechanism. Morphological changes include a reduction in autonomic neuron cell number, higher density of lipofuscin in neuronal cytoplasm and degenerative changes in the vasa nervorum. In both the sympathetic and parasympathetic systems there is evidence of reduced nerve conduction velocity. In cholinergic transmission in the parasympathetic nervous system cardiac muscarinic receptor responses decline, probably due to a reduction in receptor sensitivity to acetylcholine. More recently, evidence has come to light which indicates that the flux of calcium ions across the autonomic neuronal cell membranes is progressively impaired with age.

The net effect of these changes is reduced efficiency in the sympathetic and parasympathetic systems which reduces the ability of older people to put into effect the responses required to maintain physiological homeostasis.

Under normal circumstances this does not cause a problem to healthy elderly people but in the presence of pathological processes in effector organs, or when environmental stresses are extreme, physiological failure is likely to occur.

It is therefore possible to understand the scenario whereby an elderly person with cerebrovascular disease involving the hypothalamus and with a reduced ability to constrict peripheral blood vessels is exposed to a low environmental temperature and who might be taking, for example, a phenothiazine tranquillizer which further impairs peripheral vasoconstriction; the person is then unable to maintain a core body temperature above 35°C and lapses into hypothermia.

Impairment of thermoregulation

For the reasons outlined above, a substantial proportion of older people are unable to maintain their core body temperature within the normal range. In such people a persistent low environmental temperature may result in hypothermia, and similarly, a persistent high environmental temperature can lead to hyperthermia.

Obviously, the clinical importance of these conditions will vary in different parts of the world, though it must be pointed out that a frail elderly person with poor autonomic responses may develop accidental hypothermia on a relatively warm day.

Hypothermia

Studies in the United Kingdom have shown that during winter as many as 10% of people living at home over the age of 75 have body temperatures of less than 35.5°C when they get up in the morning. Nevertheless, severe accidental hypothermia has become less common during the 1980s and 1990s in the United Kingdom, probably as a result of increased public and professional awareness of the condition and its predisposing factors, better insulation of houses and the more widespread provision of central heating.

Many factors contribute to producing accidental hypothermia in old people and these are summarized in Box 5.1. There is evidence to show that there is blunted appreciation of cold with increasing age. There is a strong correlation between the incidence of accidental hypothermia and socioeconomic status, leading to inadequate clothing, inadequate heating and poor insulation of houses. Many old people have a diminished metabolic rate and this may be exacerbated by hypothyroidism or, for example, low-output cardiac failure.

Drugs which reduce the level of consciousness, blunt the sensing of cold or impair the vasoconstrictor response to cold are also an important factor in many patients. Alcohol abuse is underestimated as a predisposing factor to accidental

hypothermia in old age. Immobility itself may contribute, partly by reducing the amount of physical activity and therefore heat generation and partly by making it difficult for people to adjust their immediate environment to keep themselves warmer. A tendency to falls is clearly an important risk factor when a person is unable to rise from the ground in a cold room or outdoors.

Box 5.1 Some of the factors which contribute to the risk of accidental hypothermia in old age

- Cognitive impairment
- Autonomic impairment
- Hypothalamic dysfunction
- Less effective vasoconstriction
- Less effective piloerection
- Inadequate clothing
- Inadequate heating
- Immobility
- Falls
- Hypothyroidism
- Alcohol
- Drugs with vasodilator properties
- Socioeconomic deprivation

Diseases of the central nervous system, particularly cerebrovascular disease and Alzheimer's dementia, are important predisposing factors, partly by damaging the central thermoregulatory centre and partly by impairing cognition and thereby preventing the normal behavioural adjustments to a cold environment.

An outline of the thermoregulatory response is given in Figure 5.1. It can be seen that the hypothalamus is thought to act like a thermostat. Its normal setting is that of the normal core body range, though this may be set higher in the presence of pyrogens. The various peripheral mechanisms are then adjusted to maintain the hypothalamic temperature setting.

Therefore, if the hypothalamus detects that body temperature is falling below the setting, the mechanisms of piloerection, peripheral vasocon-

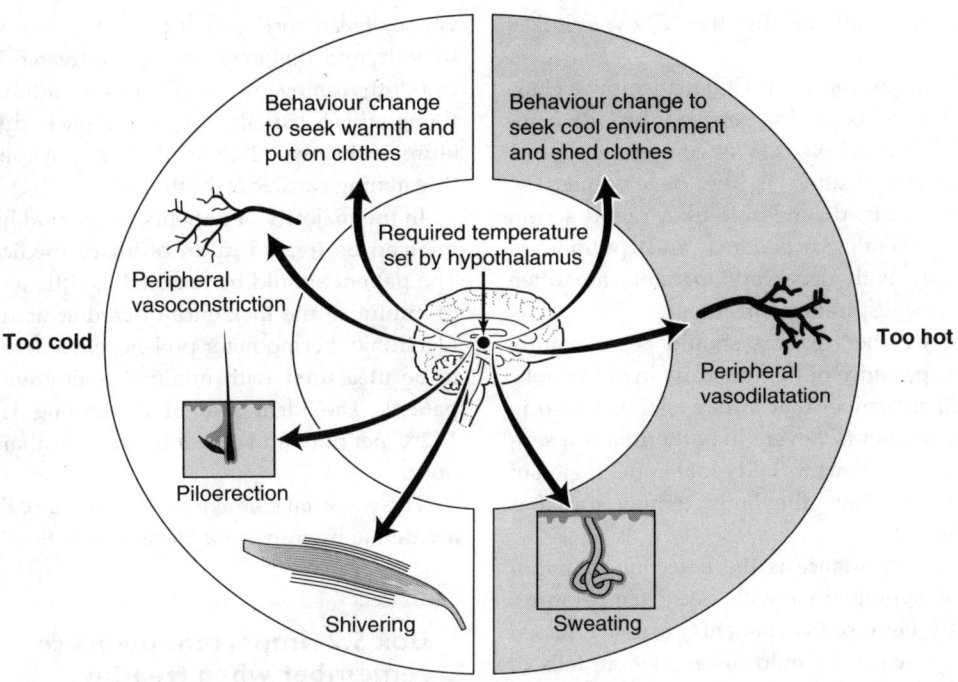

Behaviour change
to seek warmth and
put on clothes

Behaviour change to
seek cool environment
and shed clothes

Required temperature
set by hypothalamus

Peripheral
vasoconstriction

Too cold

Too hot

Peripheral
vasodilatation

Piloerection

Shivering

Sweating

Fig. 5.1 The basic elements of the thermoregulatory response.

striction and shivering will take place, and a conscious feeling of cold will make the person put on more clothes and turn up the heating. Conversely, if the hypothalamus detects that the body temperature is higher than the setting, the response will be vasodilatation, sweating, shedding of clothes and seeking out a cooler environmental temperature.

There is evidence that people who are prone to accidental hypothermia have demonstrable abnormalities in this thermoregulatory system.

In a study of survivors of accidental hypothermia who were in other ways in good health and who were compared with similar healthy elderly people who had never had hypothermia, it was demonstrated that the hypothermia survivors, when exposed to cooling of the hand, had a very poor shivering response, little reduction in hand blood flow and no change in oxygen consumption, all of which are evidence of thermoregulatory failure, whereas the normal controls responded in the normal physiological way.

Clinical features of accidental hypothermia

Accidental hypothermia is a condition in which the deep body temperature falls to 35°C or below.

It can usually be diagnosed by feeling the patient's body but it can only be established by using a low-reading thermometer. It is very important to use a thermometer which is able to detect accurately body temperatures in the low range, whether this is a traditional mercury-in-glass thermometer or a thermocouple electronic device. Core body temperature is usually measured in the rectum. Accurate readings are not likely to be obtained under these circumstances from the axilla or buccal cavity.

Hypothermic patients are pale and may show a somatic tremor, though shivering is usually absent. Consciousness may be impaired or the patient may simply be apathetic, possibly displaying disorientation, hallucinations or paranoid features. Muscle rigidity, diminished reflexes, slurred speech and occasionally extensor plantar responses are found. There is bradycardia, and respiration is slow and shallow and may be of the Cheyne-Stokes pattern.

The electrocardiogram (ECG) may show a characteristic J wave (occurring between the QRS complex and T wave), oliguria is common and one important complication is the development of acute pancreatitis, diagnosable by a raised serum amylase. Generalized oedema and pulmonary oedema may both occur and patients are often found to have respiratory infection.

In cold weather, doctors should be constantly alert to the presence of hypothermia in old people, but should remember that it may also be found in warm environments. Severe hypothermia is a serious condition, with a mortality rate in the region of 25% in those where the body temperature has fallen below 32°C.

Of equal importance is the detection of minor degrees of hypothermia with body temperatures around 34°C because such patients are easily missed and they present with mild disorientation, falls or inability to cope with looking after themselves.

Management of hypothermia

Slow rewarming is required, keeping the patient well covered with blankets in a warm room. In old age rapid rewarming has been found to increase the mortality rate, largely due to substantial falls in systemic blood pressure when extensive cutaneous vasodilatation occurs.

Cardiac monitoring is helpful to identify the frequent occurrence of cardiac dysrhythmias. These usually consist of ventricular ectopics which respond to appropriate anti-arrhythmic therapy. Clinical observations have shown that the incidence of life-threatening cardiac arrhythmias such as ventricular tachycardia and ventricular fibrillation are most likely to occur as the patient is rewarmed through the 31–33°C range.

Care must be taken that the patient does not aspirate vomit. A clear airway must be maintained and many clinicians give an antibiotic on the assumption that the patient will have a respiratory infection. Intravenous fluids must be used with great caution.

Hypokalaemia must be looked for and corrected. Hypotensive patients should be given intra-venous hydrocortisone. If patients are found to be hypothyroid this may need to be treated by using triiodothyronine in small doses intravenously, though this is usually not given if the body temperature is below 32°C as it may precipitate life-threatening cardiac arrhythmias.

In the majority of patients, accidental hypothermia can be treated in an ordinary medical ward. The patient should be handled as little as possible to minimize the incidence of cardiac arrhythmias. Electronic thermometer probes enable temperature to be measured with minimal interference to the patient. The ideal rate of rewarming is around $1/2$°C per hour and certainly not more than 1°C per hour.

The essential elements of treating a patient with accidental hypothermia are shown in Box 5.2.

Box 5.2 Important points to remember when treating accidental hypothermia in old people

- Cover patient with bedclothes and nurse in a warm, quiet room.
- Handle the patient as little as possible.
- Rewarming should be gradual, at $\frac{1}{2}$ –1 °C per hour.
- Detect and treat infection.
- Detect and correct hypothyroidism.
- Detect and treat life-threatening cardiac arrhythmias.
- Correct hypokalaemia if present.
- Give i.v. fluids very cautiously, and only if absolutely necessary.
- Look for pancreatitis.
- Remember the patient may remain thermally unstable after rewarming.

Although accidental hypothermia of a severe degree has become less common in the United Kingdom and similar countries, there is clinical evidence to suggest that mild degrees of hypothermia are still a common problem in cold weather. Prevention depends largely upon public awareness campaigns, supervision of vulnerable people by friends, relatives and statutory services, the provision of adequate clothing, housing and heating and good nutrition. People known to be particularly prone to hypothermia should be visited regularly by, for example, the district nursing service to have their body temperature checked, and may benefit from additional heating or the provision of low-voltage safety electric blankets in cold weather. It is important not to create an environmental temperature which is too high as this may result in hyperthermia in the same group of patients.

Hyperthermia

While true accidental hyperthermia is rare in temperate climates, it is known that mortality in old people peaks at the time of very high ambient temperatures.

Recent research in Malta showed a high prevalence of marginal hyperthermia in frail people living in an institution during exceptionally high environmental temperatures, during a heat wave.

Relatively simple measures, such as the provision of additional drinking water, avoidance of direct sun, appropriate clothing and the use of fans, will enable the majority of such people to maintain a normal body temperature.

Orthostatic hypotension

Autonomic dysfunction is the commonest cause of persistent postural hypotension, though there are many other causes which are outlined on page 46. Postural hypotension can be defined as a drop of 20 mmHg in systolic blood pressure (BP) or 10 mmHg diastolic blood pressure on rising from the lying to the standing position. In a young person, a transient drop of this magnitude may cause minor and fleeting symptoms of lightheadedness before the normal vasomotor regulating mechanism compensates.

If the compensatory mechanism fails as can occur in autonomic dysfunction, older people can have symptoms of postural hypotension which persist for as long as they remain on their feet. In severe cases this will lead to fainting with loss of consciousness and a collapse to the ground. In others the reduced cerebral perfusion will lead to confusion and disorientation, and falls may occur as a result of poor balance. The reflexes maintaining blood pressure are summarized in Figure 5.2.

The afferent fibres begin in the baroreceptors of the carotid sinus and then pass through the glossopharyngeal nerve to the brain-stem vasomotor centre. Efferent impulses pass through the spinal cord and the preganglionic fibres to the sympathetic chain and through postganglionic fibres to the blood vessels where their action is one of vasoconstriction. Testing this reflex at various points has shown that in the majority of old people with postural hypotension the failure is central rather than peripheral. However, impairment of the peripheral vascular smooth muscle in old age is probably an important contributing factor, and in some individuals, disease of the receptor at carotid level has been shown to be important.

The most important conditions associated with postural hypotension are shown in Box 5.3. Postural hypotension is generally seen in people who are rather frail and many of the patients have multiple pathology. Drugs are a very important contributing factor in a large number of patients, and lack of physical activity with down-regulation of the reflex is also important.

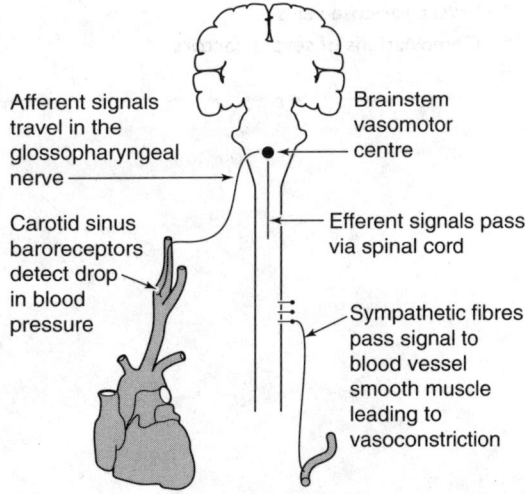

Afferent signals travel in the glossopharyngeal nerve

Brainstem vasomotor centre

Carotid sinus baroreceptors detect drop in blood pressure

Efferent signals pass via spinal cord

Sympathetic fibres pass signal to blood vessel smooth muscle leading to vasoconstriction

Fig. 5.2 The basic elements of the baroreflex maintaining blood pressure in the upright position.

The diagnosis and management of postural hypotension due to autonomic dysfunction is described along with the management of other causes of postural hypotension in Chapter 13.

Box 5.3 Factors associated with postural hypotension

- Drugs
  — antihypertensives
  — diuretics
  — anticholinergics
  — tricyclic antidepressants
  — L-dopa preparations
  — phenothiazines
  — barbiturates
- Autonomic dysfunction
  — idiopathic autonomic neuropathy
  — multisystem atrophy
  — diabetic neuropathy
  — postinfection
  — drug-induced
  — amyloidosis
- Various bacterial and viral infections
- Low cardiac output states
- Depleted blood volume
  — haemorrhage
  — dehydration
  — salt depletion
- Severe varicose veins
- Combinations of several factors

Falls

Falls are a common and important presenting symptom of disease in elderly people. Investigation and management therefore constitutes a substantial proportion of the work of specialists in geriatric medicine. Students should be fully conversant with the differential diagnosis of falls in old people, and in this chapter the important causes of falls, the features which differentiate them clinically, and investigations which help refine the diagnosis are detailed below. Before considering falls as such, the following paragraphs will deal with the important underlying concepts of sway and muscle strength.

Sway

Maintenance of the erect posture requires the balancing of a large mass with a high centre of gravity over a relatively small base. This fine balance is maintained by the antigravity muscles, with muscle activity being informed by sensory information from the skin, muscles, joints, eyes and vestibular system.

As soon as the centre of gravity begins to move away from the base the deviation is sensed and the appropriate muscles then contract to correct the movement. These complex postural reflexes are acquired in childhood, mature during early adolescence and remain unconscious throughout life in healthy individuals.

Central processing of the incoming sensory information takes place largely in the cerebellum, mid-brain and hind brain, though there clearly is an important involvement, in reflex fashion, of the motor cortex.

As with many other automatic body functions, the reflex maintenance of posture becomes impaired as people reach old age. In Figure 3.1 (see page 19), the amount of sway in relation to age is shown in the form of a graph, and it can be seen that it is at a minimum between the ages of around 15–60 and then tends to become pronounced again in people over the age of 75. Therefore, aged people are less able to correct changes in body position and in the centre of gravity quickly and adequately and this is one of the reasons why they are prone to falls.

Measurement of sway

There are several ways of measuring sway, though one of the best ways of illustrating it in an individual is to generate a 'sway' diagram, which tracks the deviation from the centre point as an individual is attempting to stand still. The spread of the sway line indicates the amount of sway taking place over a period of time.

One classical study performed by Sheldon in the 1960s used the sway diagram technique to study the change in sway in individuals of different ages. This is shown in Figure 6.1.

Similarly, individuals who are suspected of having impaired balance with excessive sway can be studied in the same way and it is possible to capture examples of extreme deviation from the centre of gravity. Such an example is shown in Figure 6.1.

Muscle weakness

Locking of the knee joints, the last movement in a series of strong muscle action in the powerful antigravity muscles of the lower limbs, also contributes

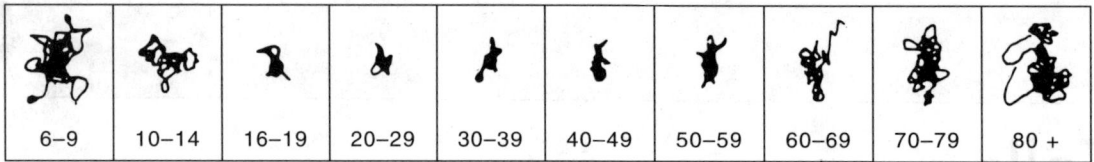

| 6–9 | 10–14 | 16–19 | 20–29 | 30–39 | 40–49 | 50–59 | 60–69 | 70–79 | 80 + |

Fig. 6.1 Sway tracings of individuals at different ages. Maximum sway is seen in the very young and very old. Very wide deviations, as seen in the 80+ group, indicate a proneness to lose balance and fall (after Sheldon 1963 Gerontologia Clinica 5:1 32).

to standing erect. While there is little evidence that loss of muscle power associated with ageing is in itself the cause of falls, it is likely that this is one of a number of predisposing factors in some old people. People with specific diseases leading to weakness in the antigravity muscles are certainly more prone to falling. Examples would include the proximal myopathy of osteomalacia, individuals with peripheral motor neuropathy, and those with excessive weakness of the lower limbs as a result of disuse when there is a painful condition of the knees or hips.

These underlying factors of excess sway and relative weakness of lower limb muscles form a backdrop against which the more refined diagnosis of the cause of falls in an individual should be interpreted.

In the context of an individual with excess sway and only just enough lower limb power to remain erect, relatively minor further impairment of, for example, coordination, will result in overt falls.

The differential diagnosis of falls

In Table 6.1 the most common causes of falls are outlined alongside some important distinguishing clinical features and important investigations. Some of these require further discussion.

Environmental causes of falls

Hazards in the immediate environment, particularly in the home, are an extremely important rea-

son for falling in old age, and yet to a great extent they can be avoided by thoughtful attention to everyday environmental objects. Examples would include inadequate lighting, and inconvenient objects such as mats, carpets and other things left lying around. Outdoors they may include uneven pavements, roads and garden paths.

Table 6.1 Some common causes of falls in old age.

Cause	Type of fall	Typical investigation
Cardiac arrhythmia	Collapse with loss of consciousness (syncope)	Electrocardiogram (ECG) 24-hour ECG
Postural hypotension	Faint	Lying and standing blood pressure
Generalized cerebrovascular disease	Loss of balance, trip, pain	Computed tomography (CT) headscan
Joint disease		Radiographs
Parkinson's disease	Loss of balance, trip	Trial of L-dopa therapy

Table 6.1 (contd) Some common causes of falls in old age.

Cause	Type of fall	Typical investigation
Vestibular disease	Vertigo, loss of balance	Tests of vestibular function
Muscle disease	Collapse, trip, weakness collapse	Electromyogram, muscle biopsy
Epilepsy	Loss of consciousnessness,	Electroencephalogram, CT headscan
Motor and sensory neuropathy	Loss of balance	Nerve conduction studies
Cerebellar disease	Ataxia, loss of balance	CT and magnetic resonance imaging
Sedating drugs	Loss of balance, drowsiness	Trial of drug withdrawal

Most falls associated with environmental hazards will result because of tripping or toppling over. It can be appreciated that younger, fitter individuals are unlikely to fall as a result of this but an elderly subject with, for example, Parkinson's disease, poor vision or a stiff painful hip would be very much at risk.

Therefore, it is very important that the clinician should always look at environmental hazards and physical impairments as synergistic causes of falls in vulnerable elderly people.

Inadequate vision

Most people with complete blindness or severely impaired sight do not fall frequently, particularly if they acquired their visual loss earlier in life. They take great care and compensate for their lack of sight, and there is some evidence that they actually trip less often than sighted people. However, frail old people who lose their vision rapidly or who have moderately impaired vision often fail to make the necessary adjustments to cope with this and are then prone to tripping, particularly when environmental hazards such as uneven floors are present.

Neurological causes of falls

There are many diseases of the central and peripheral nervous system which can result in falling, and it is helpful to look at these in two main groups: firstly, those chronic conditions which impair postural stability; and secondly, neurological impairment of sudden onset leading to abrupt cessation of normal postural stability with a fall to the ground.

Chronic neurological disease

Some patients have obvious neurological impairment and it is easy to understand why this will predispose to falling. Examples would include hemiparesis, severe Parkinson's disease, severe cerebellar dysfunction, other severe movement disorders such athetosis and chorea, gross peripheral neuropathy etc. Such patients do not present diagnostic difficulties. On the other hand, in many elderly people there are subtle changes in the same neurological systems which require careful investigation to establish the diagnosis; the physical signs may be relatively minimal and yet there is a definite predisposition to falls.

Examples of such cases would be early Parkinson's disease, subtle strokes with impairment of the processing of sensory signals, minor degrees of cerebellar dysfunction and early peripheral neuropathies. The importance of discovering such conditions in their early stage is that some may be more amenable to treatment, and, more importantly, compensation for the deficit is more easily achieved by physiotherapy and other rehabilitation methods.

Sudden neurological loss causing falls

Epilepsy. Epilepsy is relatively common in old people. In many the diagnosis is obvious: for example, in an old person who falls with a grand mal fit where there is a good witness account of what happened. Some of the common conditions of old age, such as cerebrovascular disease, dementia and cerebral tumours all predispose to epilepsy. In a grand mal convulsion a patient loses consciousness and has a classical tonic clonic convulsion, usually with incontinence. Partial seizures are more difficult to diagnose and may cause falls without loss of consciousness.

The diagnosis is worth pursuing in old people because the response to anticonvulsant therapy is as effective as in the young.

Drop attacks. As mentioned in the previous chapter, the pathophysiology of drop attacks is not fully understood. Such patients drop to the ground in full consciousness and there is often a delay before limb function and balance are regained to enable the patient to rise again.

Some such patients probably do have vascular insufficiency in the vertebrobasilar system and in a small proportion this is related to head movements, particularly turning the neck to the right or left.

Transient ischaemic attacks

Most people with transient ischaemic attacks do not fall. However, it is thought that a small proportion of patients will fall as a result of sudden unilateral limb weakness occurring as a result of a TIA in the carotid territory. It is also possible, though not proven, that some patients with drop attacks are having transient ischaemic attacks in the vertebrobasilar territory.

Cardiac causes of falls

In recent years a greater understanding has been gained of the relationship between heart disease and falling in old age. Some of the more important causes deserve specific mention in this book.

Stokes–Adams attacks

A Stokes–Adams attack is, by definition, sudden loss of consciousness due to sudden cessation of cardiac output, with spontaneous recovery.

If the patient is examined whilst still uncon-

scious there is usually no pulse or a severe bradycardia and either very low or absent blood pressure. Clearly, if the patient is standing when it occurs it is a cause of falling. A more detailed account of the dysrhythmias concerned is contained in Chapter 13. However, in the context of this chapter it is worth mentioning that the identification of conditions such as complete heart block, intermittent complete heart block, the sick sinus syndrome and the syndrome of carotid sinus hypersensitivity is important because all are amenable to treatment by the insertion of a cardiac pacemaker.

Permanent pacemaker insertion should always be made available to people with these conditions irrespective of age, and the results of treatment are extremely good.

Similarly, in patients who have Stokes–Adams attacks due to severe tachyarrhythmias, anti-arrhythmic therapy often brings the condition under control and thereby prevents falling.

Intermittent cardiac arrhythmias

If a cardiac arrhythmia is suspected as a cause or contributing factor in falls in old age, it is often necessary to try to obtain further evidence of this by performing an ambulatory electrocardiogram (ECG) test. In some patients unequivocal evidence will be obtained from the relationship between an arrhythmia and symptoms, particularly if the patient is able to record symptoms in an event diary simultaneously with having the ambulatory ECG performed.

Vascular causes of falls

Postural hypotension

As mentioned in an earlier chapter, postural hypotension is commonly found in old people and often leads to symptoms, including falls. The history often enables the clinician to distinguish postural hypotension as a cause of falling. The patient usually describes falling shortly after assuming the upright posture, particularly on getting up from bed or from the chair after prolonged rest.

In such people the blood pressure should be

measured with the patient lying down and then immediately after standing and 2 minutes after standing.

In patients with severe autonomic impairment the postural hypotension will persist in the upright position, though more commonly there will be a fall in postural systolic blood pressure for a few minutes after rising, which then improves and leaves the patient symptom-free whilst walking around. A detailed discussion on the investigation and management of postural hypotension is found in Chapter 13.

Other causes of syncope

Some of the causes of syncope have already been mentioned, namely postural hypotension and cardiac arrhythmias. However, in old age there are some other mechanisms which are worthy of spe-

cial mention, largely because they are virtually confined to old people.

Strain syncope

Some elderly people have to strain to open their bowels. This results in the Valsalva manoeuvre and the fall in blood pressure (BP) can be prolonged and then lead to patient's falling to the ground after they stand up from the toilet.

Similarly, some elderly men with prostatic hypertrophy need to strain to pass urine and the sustained rise in intra-abdominal and intrathoracic pressure results in a fall of venous return to the heart with a consequent drop in BP which leads in turn to syncope.

Thus an elderly man might complain that he frequently finds that he has fallen to the floor in the toilet and he will be particularly prone to this if he rises to pass urine at night.

Falling as the presenting feature of acute severe medical illnesses

Occasionally, a patient will fall to the ground as a consequence of a major medical catastrophe such as stroke, myocardial infarction with arrhythmia or hypotension, or gastrointestinal bleeding.

In such cases the diagnosis usually comes to light fairly quickly and the reason for the fall becomes obvious. This chapter does not contain an exhaustive and complete catalogue of the causes of falling in old age, though such details can be obtained by referring to one of the major textbooks of geriatric medicine.

In Figure 6.2 the differential diagnosis of falling in old people is illustrated graphically and this should serve as an aide-mémoire to the student who is assessing an elderly patient complaining of falls.

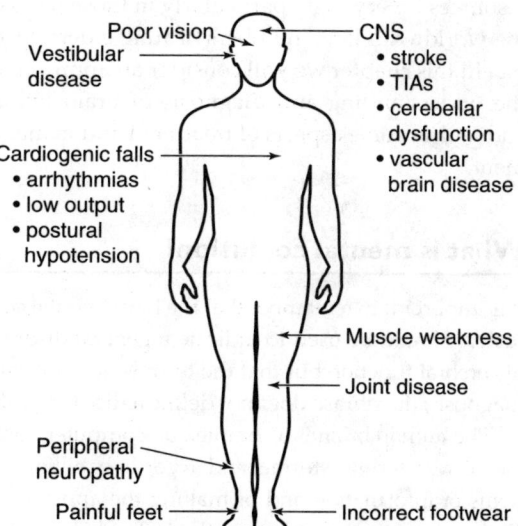

Fig. 6.2   Important causes of falling in old age.

7

Mental confusion (Brain failure)

Introduction

The assessment and management of patients with brain failure is a very important aspect of geriatric medicine. Acute confusional states have a high incidence in frail elderly people and there is a high and rising prevalence of chronic brain failure with advancing age. Acute brain failure can be provoked by a very wide variety of general medical conditions, and this can often present a considerable challenge to the clinical skills of the geriatrician. Both acute and chronic brain failure result in failure to cope, with all the social consequences which that entails. Also, the cost in terms of medical and social resources is very high, particularly in those parts of the world with large numbers of frail, elderly people. In this chapter we will consider an approach to the understanding and diagnosis of brain failure and look at some aspects of treatment and management.

What is mental confusion?

It is important to remember that the term 'mental confusion' should be used to indicate a general disorder of cerebral function but that the term is not in itself a diagnosis; the phrase does not define a disease entity.

The human brain is a complex biocomputer, capable of registering, storing and recording billions of items of information and of making the appropriate choice of action in response to them. The biochemical and physiological bases of such familiar concepts as consciousness, memory and attention are only just beginning to be understood, and even the most sophisticated of modern computers is not yet able to reproduce such phenomena. Consequently, the brain is understandably vulnerable to minor changes in the supply of various fuels, such as oxygen and glucose, or to other chemical or traumatic disturbances to its functioning units, the neurons. Understandably, when brain failure occurs it is consistently ushered in by loss of the most sophisticated function of the brain: that is, the ability to orientate it in time and place in relation to the external world and to dictate a course of action appropriate to the social framework in response to stimuli from outside.

Therefore, when this topmost function is disrupted we call the resulting state confusion; the patient is in a state of bewilderment and perplexity in which he or she cannot relate properly to either the people or the objects in the world around.

The world 'confusion' has been used for many years in the context of brain failure and the word is clearly understood by health care professionals and the public at large.

Some clinicians have criticized the use of the word 'confusion' on the grounds that it is imprecise and could be misunderstood, and some people prefer to use the term 'brain failure'.

Classification of brain failure in old age

Various classifications have been proposed and the student is referred to major textbooks of neurology and geriatric medicine for further details.

One broadly accepted approach is to subdivide brain failure into intrinsic brain failure, where there is organic brain pathology, either obvious to the naked eye or microscopically; and extrinsic brain failure, where structural brain changes are not present and the disturbance is purely one of function resulting from biochemical or physiological changes.

Intrinsic brain failure

This is usually caused by one of the primary dementias such as Alzheimer's disease, Lewy body dementia, Creutzfeldt-Jakob disease etc., or by multi-infarct dementia related to vascular changes in the brain, or to other cerebral pathologies such as brain tumours, subdural haematoma etc.

Extrinsic brain failure

This is also sometimes referred to as a toxic confusional state or acute brain syndrome. There are very many causes and some of these are listed in Table 7.1.

Table 7.1 Common causes of brain failure in old age.

1. **Intrinsic**
- Idiopathic
- Vascular
- Other organic cerebral lesions
  - tumour, primary or secondary
  - subdural haematoma
  - normal pressure hydrocephalus

2. **Extrinsic**
- Infections
  - especially pneumonia and pyelocystitis but many bacterial, parasitic and viral infections also
- Cerebral hypoxia
  - cardiac failure
  - severe anaemia
  - respiratory failure
- Carcinomatosis
- Primarily metabolic
- Hypokalaemia, hypoglycaemia, uraemia, diabetic pre-coma, water depletion, water intoxication, hepatic failure, myxoedema
- Nutritional (vitamin deficiency)
  - pellagra (nicotinic acid deficiency)
  - scurvy (vitamin C lack)
  - vitamin B_{12} and folic acid deficiency (role uncertain)
- Environmental and social
  - social upheaval or disaster
  - bereavement
  - abrupt change of environment
- Depression
  - pseudo-demented depression
- Iatrogenic
  - barbiturates, digitalis, L-dopa, alcohol and many others

Most of these will result in an acute confusional state but the same conditions can result in a subacute or even chronic picture, so there is considerable overlap between the intrinsic and extrinsic forms of brain failure in terms of chronicity.

As has been mentioned with other physiological systems, the central nervous system in frail old people is often operating close to its failure threshold, so relatively minor physiological and biochemical changes can lead to brain failure where similar changes in a young person can be compensated for and enable the subject to remain orientated.

Thus, relatively minor febrile illnesses such as urinary tract infections can result in catastrophic acute confusional states in vulnerable elderly people. This sequence of events is illustrated in Figure 7.1.

It is also important to remember that in any individual there may be several factors contributing simultaneously to an acute confusional state and the diagnosis and management must take all of these into consideration. An example of such diagnostic interdependency is shown in Figure 7.2.

Pathophysiology of intrinsic brain failure

Structural alterations in the brain consistently occur and are progressive from maturity to old age. These occur in all individuals. The brain weight falls; there is, in some areas at any rate, a large fallout of cortical neurons, and there is a steady accumulation of two microscopic lesions known as plaques, which are deposits of an amyloid-like substance, and neurofibrillary tangles. Within the neuronal cells a brown pigment, lipofuscin, accumulates. The chemical origin of these changes is not fully understood.

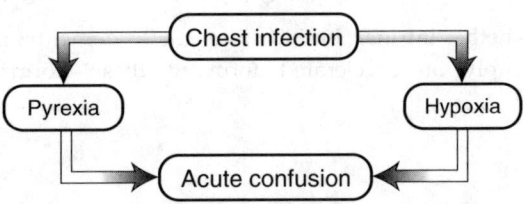

Fig. 7.1 Minor illnesses can cause acute confusion in frail old people.

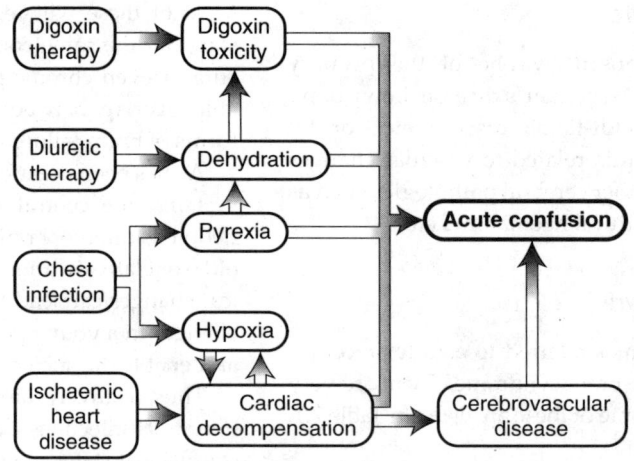

Fig. 7.2   Several factors often interact to result in acute confusion in a frail old person. This is an example; each patient will have a different mix of factors.

Changes in the production of neurotransmitters also occur with age, and recent research using sophisticated modern scanning techniques is beginning to shed some light on the functional significance of these observations.

Along with apparently normal changes in the ageing brain there are some mild losses in some aspects of mental capacity, particularly the laying down of new memory, though it must be stressed that in the healthy normal elderly brain, memory, problem-solving and abstract thinking remain very well preserved.

It is not known whether the structural changes noted in the normal ageing brain are causally related to the normal amount of functional loss. Box 7.1 summarizes some of the important aspects of the intellectual changes in old age.

Where does normal ageing end and dementia begin?

Whether intrinsic brain failure due to dementia is simply an accelerated form of these normal

---

> #### Box 7.1 Changes in intellectual function in old age
>
> * Verbal communication is well preserved.
> * The ability to lay down new memory is reduced.
> * Abstract thinking is well preserved.
> * Problem-solving is well preserved.
> * Problem-solving breaks down quickly under time pressure or when distractions impinge.

---

changes is not yet entirely clear.

However, evidence is emerging of genetic predisposition to certain forms of primary dementia, though it is likely that environmental factors will also prove to be important. Some of the rarer dementias, such as Creutzfeldt-Jakob disease and kuru, have been shown recently to be due to infection with prions.

The term 'Alzheimer's disease' was originally applied to middle-aged people with pre-senile dementia. This is a relatively rare condition. Now, the term 'senile dementia of Alzheimer's type' is usually used to describe the common form of intrinsic chronic brain failure characterized by severe cerebral atrophy and the accumulation of very large numbers of plaques and neurofibrillary tangles.

Although recent electron microscopy and histo-chemical techniques have subdivided the primary dementias into a number of discrete entities, the clinical picture does not vary a great deal and the medical and social consequences are much the same.

Another important cause of dementia is microvascular brain disease leading to multi-infarct dementia. There is now no doubt this is a separate entity from Alzheimer's-type dementia, though the two conditions, being common, frequently coexist. Patients with multi-infarct dementia show decline in cognitive function, and often also have other neurological problems such as hypertonia and hyperreflexia and a tendency to lean backwards.

A logical approach to the diagnosis of confusion

It is vital, whenever possible, to obtain information from someone who knows the patient well. Most of the really important aspects of the history need to be confirmed independently when dealing with a confused patient.

The following sequence is suggested:

1. *A detailed history of the complaint, with special reference to the rate of evolution of the mental disturbance.* Look for evidence of failing intellectual and social capacity, drug therapy, major social upheavals, coexistence of physical symptoms, previous admissions to hospital and their reasons. Ask about a history of previous mental disorder, the patient's previous personality and changes in mood.

2. *A full physical examination and observation of the patient's behaviour during the history and examination.* The range of possible diagnoses is so wide that the need for a full physical examination cannot be overemphasized.

3. *Specific investigations to confirm or refine a diagnosis which has been suspected after taking the history and examination.* For example, a computed tomogram (CT) head scan in the patient suspected of having subdural haematoma.

4. *Certain routine investigations.* Some of these have been shown to bring to light a number of important and common diagnoses which were not obvious from the history and physical examination. These include chest radiograph, electrocardiogram (ECG), full blood count, urea and electrolytes, urinalysis and thyroid function.

5. *The use of psychometric tests.* This is of little help in acute confusional states but can be extremely useful in patients with chronic brain failure, particularly when the effects are relatively subtle and when there is a need to differentiate brain failure from some of the more unusual presentations of psychiatric illness.

The onset of the illness will often be polarized into two patterns: firstly, the abrupt onset of confusion in a patient previously vigorous, mentally clear and socially independent. This suggests a symptomatic confusional state and urgently demands exclusion of an organic lesion. At the other end of the spectrum is the protracted development of odd behaviour, memory problems and failure to cope, suggesting a dementing process. This long course, can, however, eventually erupt as a social crisis and then masquerade as acute confusion.

The gradually developing mental changes can be quite subtle: minor offences against the social code, a barely perceptible fall in the standard of dress or personal hygiene, a coarsening of language or inability to handle money affairs as astutely as before.

An articulate lay person, well acquainted with the patient, will often help to distinguish between mere personal eccentricity and what is truly abnormal for the person in question. Gross evidence will often be forthcoming in the shape of aimless wandering and getting lost, progressive incompetence in self-care, hoarding, proneness to domestic accidents, and inability to use kitchen instruments safely.

The later stages of a primary dementia include profound memory loss, confabulation, false recognitions (for example, a nurse is misidentified as the patient's daughter), incontinence and convulsions. Examination at this stage may reveal dysphasia, apraxia, paratonic rigidity and total disorientation.

Drugs as a cause of confusion

A large number of drugs can cause confusion so it is important to know not only about those currently prescribed, but also about any lapsed prescriptions held in reserve at the patient's discretion, and any 'over-the-counter' drugs.

Various psychotropic drugs, sedatives, sleeping tablets, antidepressants, digoxin, antiparkinsonian drugs and antihypertensive drugs are amongst the commonest offenders in this context. It must also be remembered that alcoholism is by no means rare in old people and that elderly patients with alcoholism usually deny or play down their drinking habits. There is a tendency for young people to underestimate alcoholism as a cause of physical and mental ill health in the elderly.

Social upheavals and disasters as a cause of confusion

These include:

- bereavement
- dismissal from employment
- financial worries
- difficulties in adjusting to retirement and moving to an unfamiliar neighbourhood.

Such changes may precipitate a true confusional state if the patient is on the brink of cognitive failure or develops an underlying acute medical illness. However, such life events can also precipitate depression which may be easily diagnosed for what it is or may present as pseudodementia due to depression. This is of special importance since it is a treatable and often reversible condition with a good prognosis if it is recognized. It is easily mislabelled as dementia, because apathy and failure of attention can give a falsely poor performance on tests of intellectual ability or memory. Nevertheless, when the history is taken with care, the diagnosis can usually be made. Some of the distinguishing features between true dementia and pseudodementia due to depression are shown in Table 7.2.

Physical examination

As has been shown in Table 7.1, the conditions which can cause extrinsic brain failure, particularly in the form of an acute confusional state, cover almost the whole of internal medicine. Therefore, it would be inappropriate to list all the possible physical signs in this book.

It is important to omit nothing from the physical examination, including close examination of the head and neck, the visual fields, the ears and the pelvis.

A few particularly important points need to be mentioned here. Pneumonia is a common cause of confusion, but in the elderly, physical signs in the respiratory system are often minor or atypical or made difficult to interpret by chronic changes in

Table 7.2 Some features which distinguish dementia from pseudodementia due to depression.

Dementia	Pseudodementia due to depression
• Long time course	• Short time course
• Cognitive loss consistent	• Cognitive loss variable and selective
• Few 'don't know' answers	• Many 'don't know' answers
• Delusions unusual and inconsistent	• Negative delusions common and persistent
• Hallucinations rare	• Auditory hallucinations quite common
• Emotional responses few and variable	• Often sad and distressed
• No response to a trial of antidepressant therapy	• Responds to antidepressant therapy

the lungs and thorax, age-related changes and the presence of heart failure. Although the majority of elderly people with significant infection develop a fever, this is often missed if core body temperature is not measured properly because the level of pyrexia is often much lower than in young people with similar illnesses. In patients whose history is compatible with chronic intrinsic brain failure, there often remains a nagging doubt that there could be an underlying structural cerebral lesion, such as a tumour, abscess or subdural haematoma. Suspicion of these is legitimately raised by severe headaches, failing vision, focal neurological signs, epilepsy or a history of trauma.

Some more general features help to distinguish intrinsic brain disease from other kinds of confusion. For example, in the demented patient the use of language is poor, only simple ideas are vocalized, neologisms are common and replies to questions are often tangential. Patients will often ask for a question to be repeated in order to gain time to reply, or will answer one question by asking another.

In extrinsic confusion, on the other hand, as in an otherwise healthy person with pneumonia, there is often normal or unusually vivid use of language and its thought content is rich.

Incontinence of urine or faeces is more likely to occur in intrinsic brain failure than in other confusional states. It usually occurs at an earlier stage in multi-infarct dementia than in Alzheimer's-type dementia. Two other features of general behaviour often present in dementia are nocturnal wandering and constant restless fiddling with clothes and other objects.

Use of investigations has been discussed above.

Use of psychometric tests

A number of simple, quickly performed tests of questionnaire type are now widely used, and have been well validated against more complex psychological tests. An example of such a mental status questionnaire is given in Table 7.3. Of course, this questionnaire was validated for use in the United Kingdom and it must be remembered that such psychometric tools have a cultural bias and will need to be modified and validated separately for use in different parts of the world.

Most psychometric tests when used in this clinical context contain questions designed to measure orientation, recent memory retention and conceptual ability. The tests are easily and quickly performed and give a numerical result. While they are useful as a screening procedure for recording baseline data and for following progress when skillfully used, such tests do not discriminate with the same accuracy as a global assessment by an experienced clinician.

Table 7.3 Mental status questionnaire (shortened version of Royal College of Physicans).

Question	Score
1. Age (2 years)	0/1
2. Day (exact)	0/1
3. Time (1 hour)	0/1
4. Month (exact)	0/1
5. Year (1 year)	0/1
6. Name of hospital	0/1
7. Prime Minister now	0/1
8. Date of First World War (1914)	0/1
9. Months back (6 correct sequences)	0/1
10. 20–1 counting backwards (complete)	0/1
Total	

Borderline score 7/10

Certainly, no patient should ever be labelled demented from the results of these tests alone. It must also be stressed that these tests are for use in chronic brain failure and have not been developed or validated for use in acute confusional states.

The management of patients with confusion

The need to distinguish the more chronic, intrinsic forms of brain failure from the extrinsic acute confusional states has already been emphasized: this is the first and most important step in management. Assuming that this has been thoroughly done, management has three other elements:

1. treatment of any predisposing and contributing acute medical conditions in patients with acute brain failure, and detection and treatment of the rare but treatable forms of more chronic brain failure such as hypothyroidism and vitamin B_{12} deficiency

2. the control of disordered behaviour

3. management of the whole patient in a social environment.

The first item mentioned above will depend very much on the diagnosis and is therefore dealt with in other chapters of this book and in general textbooks of medicine and geriatric medicine. We will therefore concentrate on items 2 and 3.

Management of confused patients with disordered behaviour

Confusional states are no exception to the principle that old people are better off without drugs if their use can possibly be avoided; many mild confusional states, especially simple forgetfulness, will not need any psychotropic drug therapy. Some patients are so distressed by their acute confusional state that they require medication to relieve their symptoms.

Furthermore, some patients are at risk of damaging themselves, injuring other people or exhausting themselves if drugs are not used sensibly and judiciously for the patient's overall benefit. A large number of drugs is available for use in such circumstances and the choice will depend upon the availability, local patterns of practice and the personal preferences of clinicians.

However, before prescribing drug therapy the following points should be taken into account:

- It is better to gain experience in the use of a few established drugs rather than dabbling in a wide variety, and to gain detailed familiarity with their effects and side-effects.
- Give the chosen drug in full dosage, though it is necessary to make allowances for patients of different body size. Small doses of psychotropic medication sometimes result in a worsening of an acute confusional state.
- Patients vary in their response to psychotropic drugs so it may be necessary to adjust the dose to obtain the required amount of sedation.
- Try to avoid combinations of psychotropic medication.
- Withdraw any psychotropic medication once the cause of an acute confusional state has been remedied and the underlying condition comes under control.

- All tranquillizing drugs have side-effects, some of which are particularly important in old people. These are summarized in Box 7.2.

Box 7.2 Some important general side-effects of tranquillizer therapy in elderly patients

- Postural stability will be impaired with a greater tendency to fall.
- Phenothiazines and haloperidol can cause postural hypotension.
- Phenothiazines disturb the control of body temperature and predispose people to hypothermia.
- High doses of tranquillizers reduce respiratory drive, suppress the cough reflex and can predispose to aspiration pneumonia.
- Heavily sedated people may not eat or drink properly and therefore become poorly nourished and dehydrated.

Circumstances in which drug therapy is helpful

Nocturnal wandering and restlessness

This is probably the commonest cause of final rejection of a confused old person living with relatives. Nocturnal wandering can be frightening and creates havoc from continued sleeplessness. If aimless wandering is confined to the customary hours of sleep, the therapeutic aim is to give a hypnotic which ensures a complete night's sleep but does not leave the patient drowsy and liable to fall the next day. Two very useful hypnotic drugs with a large safety margin in this context are chlormethiazole and triclofos, though the former does sometimes cause postural hypotension. Short-acting benzodiazepines such as temazepam can be helpful, though they often have a prolonged elimination time in old people and lead to hangover effects; they can be addictive.

Very long-acting benzodiazepines such as nitrazepam should no longer be used since they have very long elimination times and cause drowsiness and postural instability during the daytime.

The recently developed fast-acting hypnotics such as zolpidem and zopiclone are also very useful, particularly since they do not have a major adverse effect on sleep architecture, with good preservation of rapid eye movement (REM) sleep, but they have a disadvantage of relatively short duration of action and are therefore of limited usefulness in patients with chronic brain failure and nocturnal wandering.

In many old people with chronic brain failure there develops a curious behaviour pattern in which confusion, agitation and restless wandering appear quite abruptly in the early evening, often at around 5–7p.m. In such patients a single dose of promazine or thioridazine in the late afternoon, followed by an hypnotic 1 hour before retiring, as described above, will often control disordered behaviour.

Daytime restlessness, agitation and hyperactivity

In some people with chronic brain failure the agitation and wandering persist, day and night. Two useful drugs under these circumstances are thioridazine and haloperidol.

Both these drugs can cause postural hypotension and disturbances of body temperature; they should be started, and their dose titrated, under close observation.

Frankly aggressive behaviour and uncontrollable restlessness with hallucinations

This is a relatively rare event in confused old people but requires effective control and sometimes intramuscular therapy. The most useful drugs are chlorpromazine and haloperidol. As mentioned above, these can cause postural hypotension and disturbances of body temperature, and all phenothiazine drugs can cause parkinsonian side-effects. Chlorpromazine occasionally causes cholestatic jaundice. Very rarely phenothiazine drugs and haloperidol will cause tardive dyskinesia, which is manifested as uncontrollable movements often of a choreiform nature and frequently involving the

face, tongue and upper body, or repetitive swinging of the leg or tapping of the foot.

This rare complication is generally seen in people who have been taking high doses of phenothiazines for long periods, but occasionally occurs after the first dose. Some old people develop morbid ideas of persecution or personal ill treatment while they are confused. They may have been paranoid for long before or the suspiciousness can simply be a reaction to an unfamiliar and therefore hostile environment during an acute confusional state.

Mild paranoid symptoms can be helped by thioridazine, though more severe symptoms will require a more powerful major tranquillizer such as trifluoperazine or fluphenazine. If the confusion is part of a pseudodemented depression, vigorous antidepressant therapy is required. Such patients often respond to a selective serotonin re-uptake inhibitor such as fluoxetine, or a tricyclic antidepressant, if some sedation is required. Elderly patients with severe depression who are resistant to drugs are often helped by electroconvulsive therapy. In such difficult cases it is advisable to involve a psychiatrist with a special interest in old-age psychiatry.

Management of the whole patient

Chronic intrinsic brain failure threatens or destroys patients' ability to organize their lives effectively for independent survival, and their management often involves placement in a suitably protected environment.

It is worth remembering that insight is usually lost early in this disease, so the patients consequently suffer less than might be imagined. However, the relatives responsible for their care may suffer greatly from the restrictions and tensions introduced into their lives.

At this stage in management the two key questions are:

- Is the patient fit to live alone and, if so, what social support will be needed?
- If not fit to live alone, where should the patient be placed?

The answers to these questions depend largely upon the degree of disability, availability of informal support, availability of medical and statutory social services, and local customs and cultures in different parts of the world. In most places the reasonable demand for institutional care far outstrips the supply. Therefore, many demented people must live in the community, where they will depend on a network of support consisting of their friends and relatives as their immediate carers, statutory social services in the form of home care, and support from specialist psychogeriatric departments, often in the form of community nurses.

This enables many demented people to manage for a long period of time before continuing to be cared for at home becomes impossible and admission to a nursing home or long-stay psychogeriatric unit becomes necessary.

Table 7.4 summarizes the main features of people with a different level of intrinsic brain failure and the levels of care they are likely to require.

Table 7.4 Degrees of intrinsic brain failure and possible social solutions.

Degree	Features	Social possibilities
Mild	Distrait and forgetful. Tends to neglect housework but can still manage primitive cooking safely. Continent, personal hygiene adequate. Aware of personal identity and own address, and can find way about neighbourhood. Conversation limited but relevant. Can make special effort for special occasions	Can survive at home if competent, devoted spouse or relative. If widowed or single will need help: neighbours, home help, meals on wheels. Support in day hospital or day centre, and occasional 'respite admission'
Moderate (no physical disability)	'Happy wandering' – gets lost outside home, does not know own address. Accident-prone: leaves gas taps on, boils kettle dry, careless with fires. Kitchen neglected. Does not buy food. Sleeps in day clothes. Often incontinent of urine	If single or widowed, not safe to live alone but may struggle on with devoted relative or spouse. If alone will need place in old people's home, home for elderly mentally infirm, or private nursing home
Moderate (with physical disability such as falls, stroke, severe arthritis)	As above but mobility limited and may be chairfast or bedfast	Not fit to live alone. If with relative will need great support, possibly frequent hospital admissions. Not suitable for residential home. Probably needs long-stay bed ultimately
Severe (no physical disability)	Gross memory defect. Total neglect of hygiene. Often incontinent. Makes no effort to cook or care for self. Conversation rambling, incoherent	Exceptional relative may cope at personal expense. Patient will need long-stay bed, probably in psychogeriatric unit
Severe (with physical disability)	As above, but chairfast or bedfast	Requires long-stay bed under care of geriatrician

Other conditions sometimes confused with dementia

We have already mentioned that pseudodemented depression needs to be differentiated from true dementia. There are two other conditions which are sometimes mistaken for dementia which deserve a mention at this stage in the chapter. The first is paraphrenia or late-onset schizophrenia, which is a form of persecutory state in which the patient has paranoid delusions, often about a neighbour. The delusions are commonly of some fear of attack such as 'passing electricity under the floor'. The condition usually occurs in people who have always led withdrawn and isolated lives. The delusions occasionally lead to noisy abuse of the neighbours or the spreading of scandal. Such patients usually continue to function very well in the community. Formal testing will reveal that they do not have dementia and their paranoid symptoms can often be controlled with modest doses of phenothiazine tranquillizers.

A rather unusual condition known as the Diogenes syndrome is one in which the external appearances are of grossly disordered behaviour characterized by living in a house which has become very dirty and cluttered with large accumulations of rubbish and sometimes enormous collections of specific items such as newspapers or milk bottles. Old people suffering from this condition often have a relatively high level of intelligence and in at least half the cases described intellectual function was otherwise normal. They do not have definite signs of any psychosis or depression. They are usually rather reclusive personalities who are not at all keen to come into hospital unless they have some definite concomitant physical disease which needs hospital treatment. Once admitted they can usually be persuaded to allow their homes to be cleaned up and after discharge they will need frequent visits by home care teams to help them keep their house in reasonable order.

8

Urinary incontinence

Introduction

Urinary incontinence is one of the most important presenting symptoms of illness in old age. As with the other cardinal presenting symptoms (falls, immobility, mental confusion and social breakdown) it is important to stress that it is a *symptom* and requires careful investigation in order to diagnose its cause. It is also an extremely disabling condition, unpleasant for the sufferer and for those with whom he or she has to live. In many cases the problem can be so intractable and distressing that an old person finds it impossible to manage any longer at home and has to move into some form of residential care. Nevertheless, there is an enormous potential for treatment by the physician who is fully aware of its possible causes and is prepared to investigate and to treat it thoroughly.

Definition

Urinary incontinence can be defined as the passage of urine against the patient's will. However, the degree of severity varies enormously from slight dampness at one extreme to regular incontinence of large volumes of urine requiring special protection or curtailing life-style at the other.

Incontinence of urine is one of a number of symptoms relating to the control of micturition which may be disordered in old age. Others include nocturnal frequency of micturition, daytime frequency and urgency of micturition. In many cases these may lead in the course of time, to incontinence.

Prevalence

The findings in prevalence surveys vary widely, largely because of differing definitions of incontinence. Of course, the prevalence would also vary depending on which population is being studied; for example, the prevalence of total incontinence in long-stay hospital wards is in excess of 70% in most surveys whereas that in residential homes is between 20% and 40%. Taking into account various surveys, the prevalence of some degree of incontinence in the United Kingdom of women living at home is between 10% and 20% and for men, between 7% and 10%.

These figures are summarized in Table 8.1.

Table 8.1 Symptoms of dysuria in a series of 557 people aged 65+ (182 male, 375 female). All figures are percentages.

	Male	Female	Total
Nocturia	70	61	64
Precipitancy	28	32	30
Urgency	14	9	10
Difficulty	13	3	7
Scalding	7	13	11
Total incontinence	17	23	20
Stress incontinence	3	12	9

Note: All of these symptoms are more common in the older age group (80+).

Causes of incontinence

Broadly speaking, the causes of incontinence fall within four main subdivisions:

1. disorders of the pelvic diaphragm
2. disorders of the urethra and bladder outlet
3. disorders within the bladder itself
4. disorders of the neurological control of micturition.

In most patients the cause of incontinence will fall into one of these categories, though sometimes two or more pathological mechanisms are present simultaneously. The main patterns of incontinence outlined in Table 8.1 can be understood in terms of these four main categories of causation.

Disorders of the pelvic diaphragm

In both sexes the bladder lies on the pelvic diaphragm (the pubococcygeus and the levator ani muscles). The bladder outlet is normally maintained with the urethra at a right angle to the bladder base by the tone of these muscles and the elasticity of the connective tissue surrounding the urethra. This angle is important in maintaining closure of the bladder outlet. The base plate muscle of the bladder (part of the detrusor muscle) tends to maintain the internal urethral meatus closed as long as the base plate is flat, but as soon as the right angle of the bladder outlet is lost, the base plate muscle loses it effect in maintaining closure of the internal urethral meatus; instead it contributes towards the contracting bladder (see Fig. 8.1).

In normal micturition this process is initiated by contraction of longitudinal muscle fibres running from the bladder into the urethra which pull open the internal urethral meatus and dislocate the base plate.

When the pelvic diaphragm muscles are weak, as is the case in women with any degree of uterine prolapse, then this will lead to urethral sphincter incompetence and thus to genuine stress incontinence. Stress incontinence may also occur in women who do not show the presence of prolapse or a cystocele and it may be that in such women, incompetence of the bladder outlet is associated with changes in the elastic fibres, which help to maintain urethral closure. The external urethral sphincter is not an important muscle in the maintenance of continence, although it is useful in stopping micturition in mid-stream. Nor is there a separate anatomical internal urethral sphincter, although some muscle fibres from the detrusor muscle of the bladder which continue into the urethra have something of a sphincteric effect. Closure of the bladder outlet is very much a result of the firm supporting tissues around the urethra, together with the closing effect of the base plate and the tone of the pelvic diaphragm.

In incompetence of the pelvic diaphragm, or of the tissues surrounding the urethra, there is funnelling of the bladder outlet which leads to effective shortening of the female urethra (see Fig. 8.2).

In this condition any sudden rise in intravesical pressure would cause immediate leakage of urine, and this is referred to as stress incontinence. Genuine stress incontinence is the commonest cause of urinary incontinence in women. Although it usually occurs after childbirth it may effect nulliparous women when there is congenital weakness of the support to the urethra. It may also be due to pelvic surgery or postmenopausal atrophy and is exacerbated by anything which increases intra-

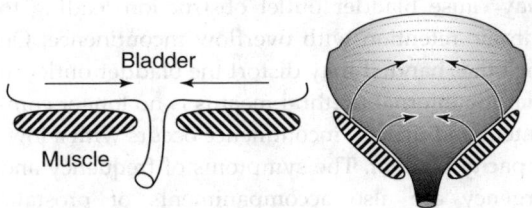

Bladder

Muscle

Fig. 8.1 The base plate of the bladder.

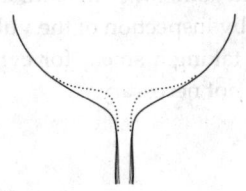

Fig. 8.2 Funnelling of bladder outlet and shortening of urethra (_ _ _ _ = normal outline).

abdominal pressure such as a mass, chronic cough or constipation.

Women with genuine stress incontinence almost invariably complain of the symptom of urinary leakage associated with physical exertion with or without frequency, urgency or prolapse.

The diagnosis of genuine stress incontinence is made largely on the history. Examination of the vulva may reveal a degree of cystocele and leakage may be seen when the patient is asked to cough, particularly in the standing position.

Occasionally it is necessary to perform a micturating cystogram to demonstrate the anatomy of the bladder outlet and indicate small degrees of incompetence of the internal urethral meatus.

Some patients with true detrusor instability, also known as unstable bladder, also sometimes complain of incontinence following cough or movement, and this can lead to confusion about the diagnosis if it is mistaken for stress incontinence. Detrusor instability is discussed later in this chapter. However, the important difference is that in stress incontinence only a small amount of urine leaks out while intravesical pressure is raised, whereas in the patient with detrusor instability a cough or movement fires off a bladder contraction which may cause considerable emptying.

Treatment of stress incontinence

In the first place, treatment of stress incontinence involves referrals to a physiotherapist who will teach the patient pelvic floor exercises to strengthen the muscles of the diaphragm and improve the performance of the sphincter. It is only when physiotherapy fails to improve the symptoms that referral to a gynaecologist or urologist should be considered.

Disorders of the urethra and bladder outlet

Women

In the female the most important condition is senile vaginitis. The lining of the adult female urethra is stratified squamous epithelium, as is that of the vagina, and it is oestrogen-sensitive, whereas the bladder epithelium is transitional epithelium and is not oestrogen-sensitive. As women grow older, stratified squamous epithelium extends in many individuals on to the trigone of the bladder. Being oestrogen-sensitive, the epithelium becomes cornified during the menstrual cycle and in times of oestrogen deprivation it becomes atrophic. This is the condition seen in senile vaginitis and similar changes may affect the urethra and indeed the trigone.

These in turn cause frequency and urgency of micturition and sometimes incontinence. The diagnosis is made by inspection of the vulva and can be confirmed by taking a smear for cytology, though this is usually not necessary.

Treatment

Oestrogen replacement orally or the use of oestrogen creams locally is often effective. Oestrogens by mouth are preferable since local application may introduce secondary infection in elderly women in whom perineal hygiene is a problem. The patient must be warned of possible breast swelling and fluid retention. Abrupt withdrawal of oral oestrogens can cause vaginal bleeding. Many clinicians now prefer to use cyclical hormone replacement therapy rather than unopposed oestrogen replacement in such patients. This also reduces the risk of endometrial cancer.

Elderly men

In this group of patients the main lesion is enlargement of the prostate. Benign prostatic hypertrophy may cause bladder outlet obstruction leading to chronic retention with overflow incontinence. On the other hand, it may distort the bladder outlet so that the internal urethral meatus is no longer competent and urinary incontinence occurs with a low-capacity bladder. The symptoms of frequency and urgency are also accompaniments of prostatic hypertrophy. Malignant disease of the prostate can cause similar symptoms.

Treatment

Selective alpha 1 blocking agents such as prazosin and indoramin can be very helpful by relaxing the smooth muscle component of prostatic obstruction. Some patients will require per-urethral partial resection of the prostate gland. In elderly men there is often more than one reason for difficulties with micturition so the results of operation can be disappointing if there is an accompanying neurogenic cause for incontinence.

Faecal impaction

A common cause of urinary incontinence in both sexes is impaction of faeces. The impacting pelvic mass may either cause incontinence with a low-capacity bladder or chronic retention with overflow incontinence. When the faecal impaction is treated, urinary and usually faecal incontinence will improve or disappear. This is a very important treatable cause of incontinence which should always be looked for and dealt with.

Disorders of the bladder itself

Almost any intrinsic disease of the bladder may reveal itself as incontinence or with symptoms of urgency, and nocturnal and daytime frequency. These include, particularly, carcinoma and the presence of a calculus. These two possibilities must always be considered and particularly suspected if microscopic haematuria is detected.

The diagnosis requires cystoscopy but this is a straightforward procedure, particularly in females, where it is easily performed as a day case. Another much more common disorder of the bladder which may cause these symptoms is cystitis.

On the other hand, the urinary infection may indicate a chronic bacteriuria, which itself may be secondary to underlying disease within the bladder or of the neurological control of micturition. These may be associated with a degree of residual urine.

In such a case the symptoms of incontinence are those of the underlying cause of bladder dysfunction, and the infection is secondary. The elimination of the infection will not then affect the symptoms. In this case there is almost certain to be recurrence of the infection, either with the same or with a different organism, within a matter of weeks or months. It is not always easy to distinguish between these two types of infection and if there is any doubt then a course of the appropriate antibiotic should be given as a therapeutic trial.

In summary, a urinary infection is occasionally the cause of incontinence. More often, the infection is a chronic bacteriuria and both it and the incontinence are evidence of another underlying pathology.

Impairment of the neurological control of micturition

This is the most important cause of incontinence in old people. Its full understanding requires an appreciation of how the young baby acquires control of micturition. A simplified account of this is as follows. In the young child the bladder fills from the kidneys. The bladder is a compliant organ and fills with minimal rise in pressure but once it distends beyond a certain point its stretch receptors are activated.

These discharge impulses through the afferent autonomic nerves to the second, third and fourth sacral segments of the spinal cord. In this area, through the various interneurons, the physiological mechanisms of recruitment and after-discharge lead to the activation of efferent impulses. These pass, from time to time, through the parasympathetic nerves causing small intrinsic contractions of the bladder wall.

As the bladder becomes more distended these contractions become more frequent until a very large one occurs which causes the bladder to empty. This emptying is reflex and the baby is therefore incontinent. The basic anatomy is shown diagrammatically in Figure 8.3.

As time goes by, the young child learns first of all to appreciate in consciousness the sensation of bladder distention by developing pathways through the lateral columns of the spinal cord to an area of the frontal cortex lying within the cingulate gyrus. At the same time the child becomes aware of the social desirability of acquiring continence.

This is a complex process which may be interrupted at a number of different levels within the central nervous system. The different lesions which cause such disruptions cause the various types of neurogenic incontinence.

Classification of neurogenic incontinence

Various classifications have been devised, though for practical purposes the student needs to understand four main categories of neurogenic bladder: the autonomous, the atonic, the reflex and the uninhibited. These are illustrated diagrammatically in Figure 8.4.

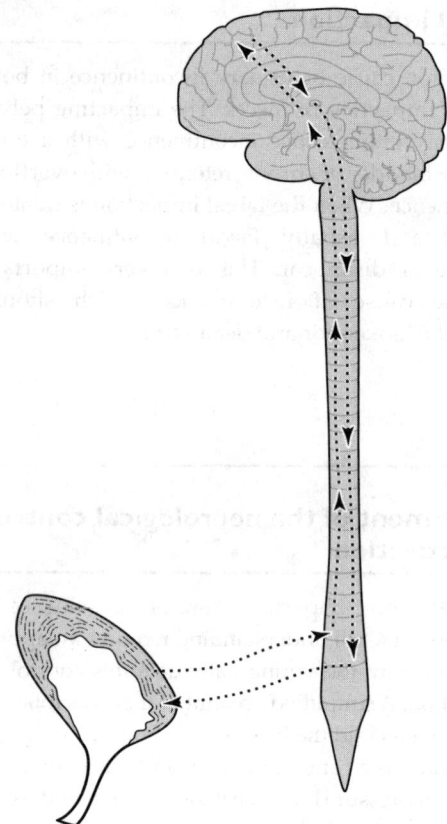

Fig. 8.3 The neurological control of micturition.

The young child, therefore, sends down through the developing long tracts in the lateral parts of the spinal cord impulses which block the reflex arc at the sacral level.

These are inhibitory impulses since they effectively inhibit the reflex of micturition. Once the child has learnt to inhibit these its bladder will fill up without emptying itself reflexly. When time and place are appropriate for micturition the child can stop inhibiting and indeed can facilitate bladder contractions, at the same time relaxing the striated muscle of the pelvic diaphragm, and also deliberately increasing intra-abdominal pressure. The child will then micturate consciously. Once this neurological process has been acquired it normally stays with the individual throughout life. The bladder of the normal adult shows no intrinsic contractions until voluntary emptying begins.

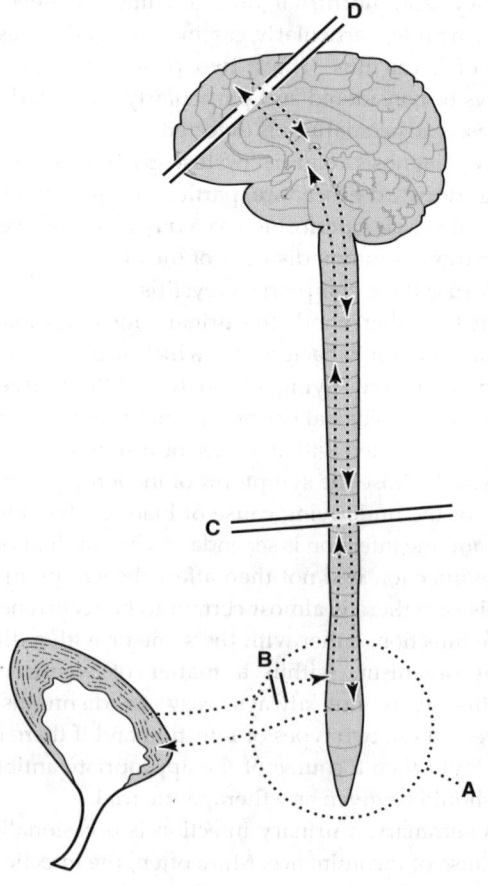

Fig. 8.4 Classification of the neurogenic bladder. A = autonomous; B = atonic; C = reflex; D = uninhibited.

The autonomous neurogenic bladder

The autonomous neurogenic bladder occurs when the bladder centre in the sacral cord is destroyed and the bladder is completely decentralized. This happens in spina bifida and very occasionally in people who have tumours of the cauda equina, or who have vascular damage to the lower end of the spinal cord. In this case the bladder will be quite devoid of conscious sensation. It will fill and empty inefficiently and automatically as a result of simple axonal reflexes and other reflex activity through the peripheral nerves. The patient will therefore be incontinent. Most patients of this type require management with an indwelling urinary catheter.

The atonic neurogenic bladder

In patients with this condition there is disease affecting the posterior nerve roots or the posterior horn cells. The sensation of bladder distention is lost although cortical voluntary inhibition is retained.

This is the typical bladder of diabetic neuropathy and will also be seen by clinicians in parts of the world where tabes dorsalis is still prevalent. Because the person is unaware of bladder distention, the bladder becomes overdistended from time to time, and gradually becomes chronically atonic. This leads to chronic retention and overflow incontinence. A similar clinical picture may also result from motor paralysis, especially as a side-effect of drugs with anticholinergic properties, and can also be the consequence of chronic bladder outlet obstruction in elderly men with prostatic hypertrophy. The management of atonic neurogenic bladders almost always requires the use of an indwelling catheter.

The reflex neurogenic bladder

This neurogenic abnormality of micturition results from a lesion above the sacral cord affecting both afferent and efferent fibres. This occurs most commonly with transection of the spinal cord due to trauma, particularly road traffic accidents. Partial lesions may result from the demyelination plaques of multiple sclerosis and impingement of osteophytes in spondylosis.

It is, therefore, the bladder of the paraplegic or paraparetic patient and it is similar to the bladder of a baby. There is neither sensation of bladder distention nor the ability to inhibit intrinsic bladder contractions, and so bladder emptying is reflex and the patient is incontinent. Occasionally, paraplegics learn to fire off intrinsic bladder contractions at a time which is suitable to them by stimulating the skin within the second, third and fourth sacral dermatomes. Since a complete synchronous relaxation of the external urethra sphincter with detrusor contraction requires intact connection to the hind brain, sometimes referred to as the pontine micturition centre, bladder emptying in the reflex neurogenic bladder is often incomplete as a result of detrusor sphincter dysynergia, and an increase in residual urine volume results.

The uninhibited neurogenic bladder

This is an extremely important cause of incontinence in elderly people. It is common and causes great distress to patients and their carers, yet in many cases a considerable amount can be done to alleviate the symptoms.

In this type of neurogenic bladder the sensation of bladder distention is retained but the power to inhibit is lost and this is typically due to a lesion in the cerebral cortex. It most commonly occurs in patients with cerebrovascular disease, including some with stroke and occasionally with cerebral tumours. It also occurs in normal pressure hydrocephalus, which tends to present with the triad of incontinence, gait disorder and mental confusion.

Some impairment of the cortical bladder centre results from ageing within the neurons of the cerebral cortex. Just as memory impairment, an increase in sway, some impairment of the control of the vasomotor function and thermoregulation may be accompaniments of ageing of the brain, so some degree of the uninhibited neurogenic bladder may be present also for this reason.

The uninhibited neurogenic bladder may be present without causing incontinence, but with the symptoms of nocturnal frequency and urgency. Since sensation is retained the feeling of desire to void often occurs when intravesicle pressure rises in association with an uninhibited contraction;

since this contraction may quickly lead to bladder emptying the patient suffers from urgency.

This type of incontinence is sometimes therefore described as urge incontinence. Clearly, patients with poor mobility are more likely to be incontinent if they suffer such urgency of micturition. In old people the uninhibited neurogenic bladder is often a predisposing cause or factor causing impairment of bladder control which can be compensated for by adjusting the environment to suit the badly functioning bladder. Thus a bedside commode or nearby lavatory allows the person with nocturnal frequency and urgency to empty the bladder safely. Such a patient may also curtail journeys out during the day to those which the badly functioning bladder can cope with. The patient may not, therefore, become incontinent unless some additional precipitating factor comes along. Usually this is some-thing which makes the patient dependent on other people. They in their turn may not realize how the bladder works and how it needs to empty quickly once the sensation of bladder distention arises.

Common precipitating factors are:

- becoming bedfast due to an acute medical condition, such as pneumonia, or due to trauma, such as fractured femur
- occasionally a change of environment, so that the old person wakes up bewildered in the night, not knowing where the toilet is
- in the context of acute brain failure
- the use of powerful diuretics.

It is essential that all nursing staff who look after the elderly are aware of the possible precipitating causes of incontinence and can take the necessary steps to minimize their impact on the patient.

Assessment and diagnosis of incontinent elderly patients

A scheme for the assessment and management of elderly people with incontinence is shown in Figure 8.5.

History and examination

A careful history should be taken and notes should be made of daytime and night time frequency, whether or not there is accompanying urgency, change in urinary stream and any sensation of incomplete emptying. Social and environmental factors should not be overlooked.

The examination should include the abdomen for a palpable bladder. Neurological examination of the lower limbs may show evidence of spinal cord disease. Rectal examination should be performed in men with symptoms suggesting prostatic disease, and in all elderly people with constipation to rule out faecal impaction.

In women, especially those suspected of having genuine stress incontinence, a vaginal examination should be performed.

Noninvasive investigations

The extent of a patient's incontinence can often be assessed from diaries which record frequency and even volume of incontinence. The time and volume of urine at each normal void is recorded together with each episode of incontinence. This provides a reasonably objective insight into the problem for the doctor, nurse, continence advisor and the patient. A mid-stream urine culture is an essential first step since adequate assessment of dysfunctional lower urinary tract states can only be carried out successfully in the absence of infection. The urine should also be tested for the presence of glucose and red blood cells.

Urodynamic tests

Most elderly people with incontinence do not require urodynamic measurements. In most individuals the type of incontinence can be diagnosed from the history and physical examination. Some

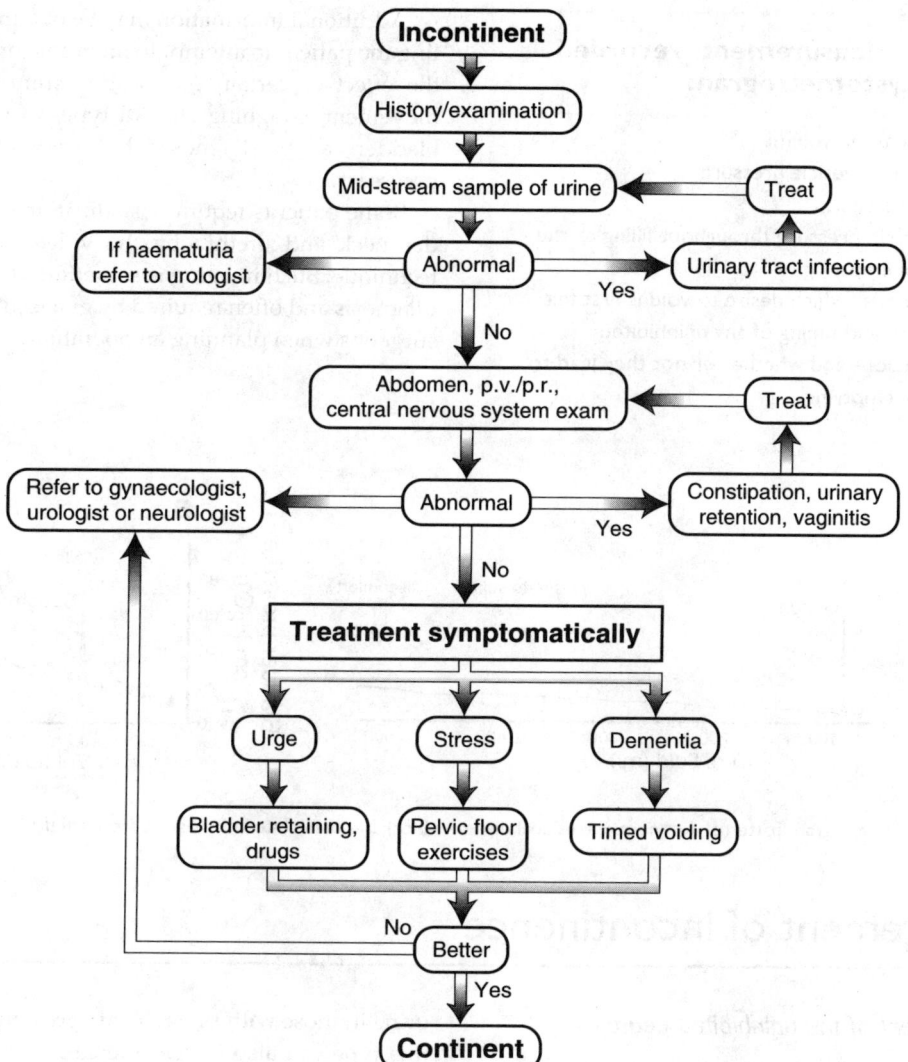

Fig. 8.5 Scheme for managing urinary incontinence in elderly people.

patients with an uninhibited neurogenic bladder require a cystometrogram to confirm the diagnosis. A cystometrogram is simply a method of observing and recording the reaction of the bladder to increasing distention. Examples are shown in Figure 8.6.

The bladder is filled from a reservoir through a two-way catheter, the other tube of the catheter being connected to a manometer and usually through that to a recording device. Often the manometer is omitted and a transducer is used to convert changes in fluid pressure to a recording on paper. The bladder is filled either with liquid or carbon dioxide. Box 8.1 lists the measurements which can be recorded by the cystometrogram.

Box 8.1 Measurements recorded by the cystometrogram

1. Residual urine volume
2. Resting intravesicle pressure
3. Bladder capacity
4. Intravesicle pressure throughout filling to the point of emptying
5. The point at which desire to void is first felt
6. Presence and timing of any uninhibited contractions and whether or not they lead to bladder emptying.

Additional information may be obtained by getting the patient to attempt to micturate or by noting the effect of certain provocative stimuli such as movement, coughing etc. All types of neurogenic bladder can be diagnosed by cystometrogram if necessary.

Some patients require visualization of the bladder neck and urethra by the video urodynamic technique. Such imaging is sometimes required for diagnosis and often required by gynaecologists and surgeons when planning an operation.

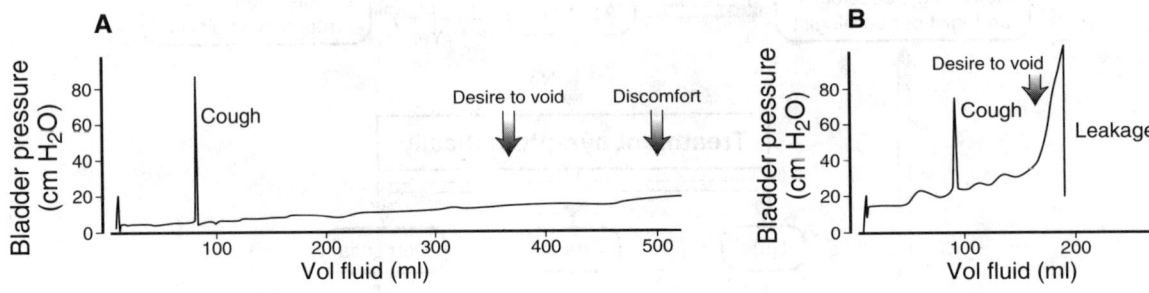

Fig. 8.6 Cystometrogram patterns. A = normal (residual urine < 10 cc); B = uninhibited neurogenic (residual urine > 10 cc).

Management of incontinence

Management of the uninhibited neurogenic bladder

The rationale for drug treatment in patients with bladder hyperreflexia due to an uninhibited neurogenic bladder is to give medication which lessens detrusor overactivity by blocking parasympathetic transmission. Drugs with an anticholinergic action, such as oxybutynin, are generally effective. The most common side-effect is a dry mouth and some patients complain of blurred vision. Occasionally, patients develop cardiac dysrhythmias and care needs to be taken in people with glaucoma.

The treatment is generally used in elderly women, and can be used in elderly men though there is a risk of precipitating acute retention of urine in those with prostatic hypertrophy. Drugs of this type can also increase residual urine volume by promoting a tendency to chronic retention and this can then cause incontinence due to overflow. It is important to tailor the time of administration of such drugs properly to meet the patient's needs.

If the patient is incontinent only at night then the medication should be given before retiring to bed, and in many cases may not need to be given at any other time. It is important that the patients are encouraged to pass urine regularly so as to keep their bladder volume well below that which precipitates an uninhibited detrusor contraction. A 2- or 3-hourly toileting regimen is often suitable.

Many patients would rather be woken at night

by an alarm clock to pass urine than be incontinent into the bed. Patients who are incontinent throughout the day should receive regular anticholinergic cover and regularly timed toileting around the clock. Patients should not have their fluid restricted though they may need to avoid taking large volumes of fluid last thing at night if they suffer from frequent nocturnal incontinence.

It must be remembered that it is vital to ensure that those patients with urgency and incontinence are as mobile as possible and that a toilet is nearby and easily accessible. In many cases this will dramatically reduce the number of episodes of actual incontinence.

Management of true detrusor instability

The management is similar to that of the uninhibited neurogenic bladder, and indeed many clinicians still use these terms loosely and interchangeably. In patients with detrusor instability, intrinsic bladder contractions may be fired off during simple bladder filling, though more often they occur as the result of a provoking stimulus which causes a sudden rise in intra-abdominal pressure, such as coughing, running or jumping. The term 'true detrusor instability' describes a condition in which there is no overt neurological disease causing failure of normal inhibition of micturition.

The cause is not really understood, though there may be a functional or even psychosomatic element to it. Patients often complain of a mixture of urge incontinence and stress incontinence. Some patients undoubtedly benefit from anticholinergic drugs and bladder drill which is described in detail below.

Bladder drill. This is a form of behavioural therapy in which patients are taught to empty their bladder regularly by the clock. They start at 1- or $1\frac{1}{2}$-hour intervals and over a period of days increase this by half an hour at a time until they can achieve $2\frac{1}{2}$-$3\frac{1}{2}$-hour emptyings. Sometimes hospital admission is used to reinforce the procedure. Bladder drill is often successful in the management of patients with true detrusor instability and can be helpful in patients with an uninhibited neurogenic bladder.

The practical management of incontinence

The differential diagnosis of urinary incontinence and an approach to its investigation and treatment are shown in Figure 8.5 (see p. 69).

Transient incontinence is often the result of systemic disorder and should clear up when the underlying medical problem has been adequately treated. Established incontinence is usually a major presenting symptom requiring specific investigation and therapy. In the majority of cases this will control the incontinence. Occasionally, however, patients with intractable incontinence present in whom no treatment is successful. This is particularly the case in patients with vascular dementia, though it may also be seen in people with Alzheimer's disease, stroke, brain tumour and some other conditions. In these cases consideration must be given to the use of pads, appliances and catheters.

Incontinence pads

Many large incontinence pads are on the market for use on beds or chairs. These contain materials which absorb liquid and they have a waterproof backing.

Unfortunately, they remain wet as the patient lies or sits on them and may thus lead to the formation of urine rashes on the skin. Also with large quantities of urine they tend to form a lake and the urine may run off the edge of the pad, wetting the bed. However, as a method of protection of bedding against the occasional wetting they have a place.

There is now a range of excellent incontinence pads designed to be worn on the person, and most of these consist of pads which are either worn in a special pair of close-fitting pants containing a pouch or fitted inside elasticated stretch pants. These are illustrated in Figures 8.7 and 8.8.

Appliances

Male. Sheath urinals are worn over the penis and are connected by tubing to a drainage bag worn on the leg. They are useful for men who are

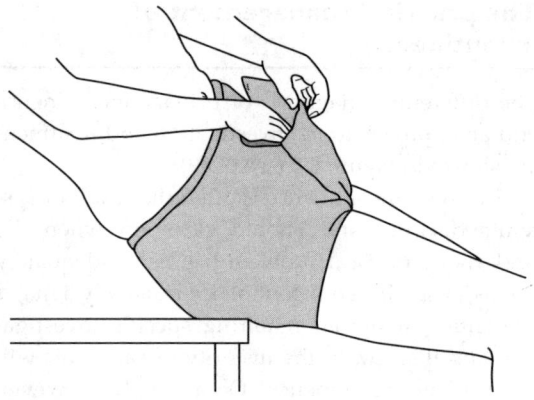

Fig. 8.7 The Marsupial pad.

bedfast because of paralysis or coma, as well as the ambulant.

Patients who are agitated or confused tend to pull sheath urinals off the penis. Various types of penile clamps are available but their use is extremely limited, and they are particularly contraindicated in patients with uninhibited neurogenic bladders, since anything which obstructs the outflow of urine during the uninhibited contraction will cause a sharp rise in intravesicle pressure, encouraging the formation of bladder diverticula and ureteric reflux.

There is a wide range of other devices on the market, some of which are suited to particular individuals. For example, the pubic pressure urinal is useful for men who are mobile and incontinent. However, it requires very accurate fitting and the patient needs to have normal cognitive function and good manual dexterity to use it properly.

Female. Although a variety of urinals designed to be worn on the body have been marketed for use with women there is none which is successful at the present time.

Catheters (men and women)

If all other methods of treatment of urinary incontinence fail then the use of an indwelling catheter to be worn permanently is the final method of control. It is not unusual for patients to prefer wearing a catheter to being continually incontinent. For this purpose, Foley catheters, retained in the bladder by an inflatable balloon, are used and they are attached to a collecting bag which is worn on the body. There are several special belts available for

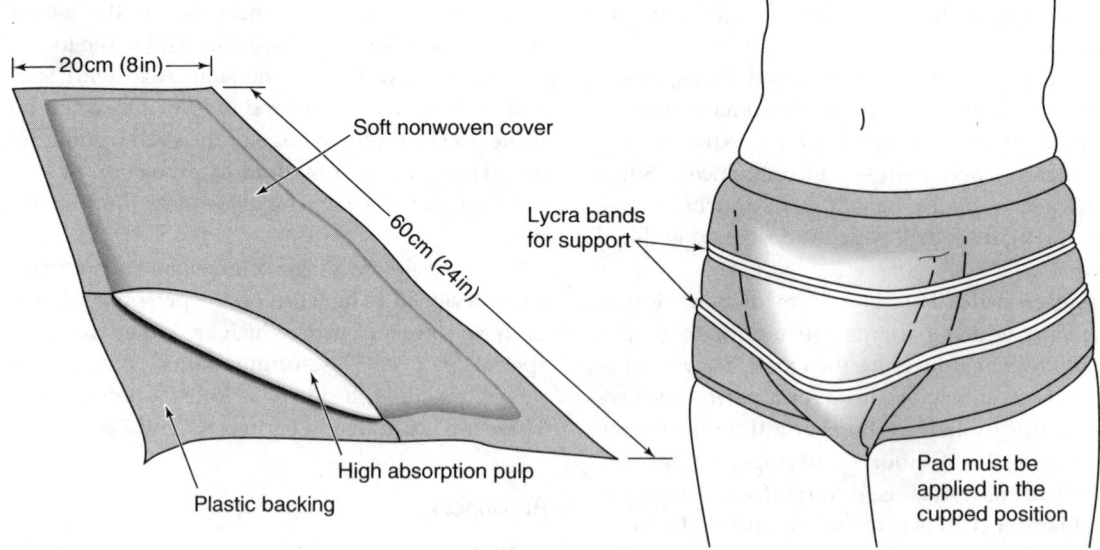

Fig. 8.8 The Maxis-plus system (Molnlycke). Loosely knitted Helanca stretch nylon pant. One size to fit waist 45–137 cm (18–54 inches).

use with disposable urine bags. On no account should an indwelling catheter be worn with a bag which either lies on the floor or is attached to the furniture, since not only is this degrading for the patient but it also tends to discourage mobility.

Leg- and body-worn bags should have a flutter valve incorporated into them so that they may also be worn when the patient is lying in bed. Patients can usually be taught to empty the bag themselves every 4–6 hours. Modern Foley-type catheters are produced with smooth, nonwettable surfaces which cause minimal damage to the urethra and also prevent adherence of salts and debris. Such catheters can be worn for periods of 3–6 months without changing, though this varies from person to person.

Latex catheters are now used for very short-term catheterization and should never be used for more than 2 weeks.

Catheters and urinary infection. One drawback with indwelling catheterization is that it is inevitably accompanied by bacterial contamination of the urine. Bacteria will ascend not only within the catheter but also in the film between the catheter and urethra. While it is possible to maintain a sterile closed system of catheter drainage for a few days it is not praticable to do this for longer periods, particularly in patients who are mobile. Therefore, bacterial contamination of the urine has to be accepted as an inevitable feature of indwelling catheterization.

Fortunately, such infection appears to be benign inasmuch as it does not produce systemic effects. In the short term, up to about 5 years, it seems to produce no serious effects on the kidney, although in the long term renal infection and its complications do occur. Since the life expectancy of most patients with intractable incontinence who may require indwelling catheterization is likely to be less than 5 years, the risk of infection can be quite reasonably accepted, particularly if by the use of an indwelling catheter it is possible for an old person to remain dry rather than be continually wet for these last years, and possibly to live at home rather than in some form of residential care.

Use of antibiotics. It is not usual practice to give antibiotics systemically in patients with indwelling catheters simply because of a positive bacterial culture from a catheter specimen of urine. Antibiotics will sterilize the urine only for a short period, then recolonization will occur. Furthermore, excessive use of antibiotics in this way will produce resistant organisms. On the other hand, if evidence of systemic infection is present in the form of fever or leucocytosis, or if the urine becomes blood-stained or has a high proportion of white cells, it is then necessary to give antibiotic therapy, preferably based on the results of urine culture.

Some patients will develop a transient bacteraemia or even septicaemia at the time of catheterization, which will require antibiotic therapy.

Bladder washouts. There is some evidence that regular bladder washouts with an acidifying solution are helpful in patients whose catheters tend to block from encrustation with crystal, though this is not necessary in the majority of patients. If there is a heavily infected sediment, washout with chlorhexidine solution can be used.

Intermittent self-catheterization. Some patients with chronic urinary retention with an atonic bladder and some patients with a reflex bladder can maintain continence by learning to pass a catheter to empty their bladder.

The catheter is immediately removed. This technique is suitable only for female patients who have sufficiently good cognitive function to learn the technique and apply it properly, and sufficiently good eyesight and manual dexterity to perform the procedure safely and effectively.

9

Faecal incontinence

Introduction

Faecal incontinence is sometimes thought of as an inevitable consequence of ageing. However, as with pressure sores, it might more appropriately be regarded as a failure of medical and nursing management; for with proper diagnosis and treatment, faecal incontinence in old people is almost entirely preventable. Its importance lies not only in the unpleasant and degrading situation in which the patients find themselves, but also in the fact that it may be a symptom of serious and possibly treatable disease of the lower bowel or elsewhere.

The effect of ageing

Ageing is associated with changes which may predispose to faecal incontinence, though not actually cause it. There is a diminution in anal squeeze pressure, due to changes in the external sphincter, which is more common in women and may be a long-term effect of childbirth. The volume of rectal distention causing desire to void diminishes in old people.

Furthermore, some elderly people have difficulty in distinguishing between fluid and flatus in the anal canal. These factors probably predispose elderly people to becoming incontinent in the presence of other causative factors.

Clinical presentation

Clinically, faecal incontinence may present in two ways: in the first place as frequent or almost constant soiling with semiformed faeces, and in the second place as the passage of a formed stool once or twice a day into the bed or clothing. These different modes of presentation have different causes and are important clues as to the diagnosis.

Causes of faecal incontinence

The causes are summarized in Box 9.1.

Box 9.1 Causes of faecal incontinence in elderly people

1. Constipation with faecal impaction and overflow incontinence
2. Colo-rectal disease
   — colo-rectal cancer
   — diverticular disease
   — inflammatory bowel disease
3. Incontinence due to diarrhoea
   — drug-induced, e.g. laxatives
   — gastric and small bowel disorder, e.g. malabsorption
   — irritable bowel syndrome
   — gastrointestinal infection
4. Neurogenic incontinence – due to loss of cortical inhibition in dementia
5. Anal sphincter defects, with or without rectal prolapse
6. Factors relating to access to toilets and handling clothing, in association with impaired mobility

---

Ano-rectal continence mechanisms

There are three important mechanisms maintaining secure closure of the anal canal. These are:

1. the ano-rectal angle, which is maintained at less than 100° by the sling-like effect of the puborectalis muscle (see Fig. 9.1)
2. the external anal sphincter, which protects especially in the face of a sudden rise of intra-abdominal pressure, for example on coughing
3. the anus itself, by its flutter valve effect, by its smooth muscle and by the conformity of the mucosal folds to each other.

Faecal incontinence due to constipation

In immobile elderly people, particularly those living in institutions, the most important cause for faecal incontinence is secondary to faecal impaction.

The patients and their carers usually complain of frequent or constant soiling of clothes and bedclothes by semi-solid faeces. The constipating mass lies at the anal verge, thereby dislocating the ano-rectal angle (see Fig. 9.2) and blunting the patient's

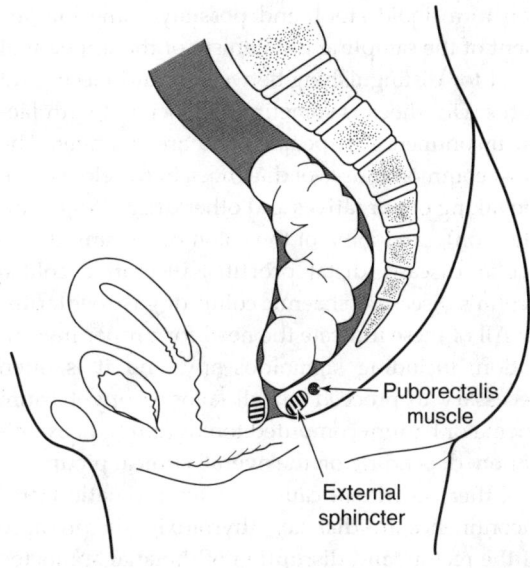

Fig. 9.2 Constipated mass dislocating ano-rectal angle.

sensory ability to discriminate between fluid, flatus and faeces. Semi-solid stool may then leak out, causing incontinence due to faecal retention with overflow. The diagnosis is made on the history and also on rectal examination. Faecal impaction by hard masses is a common cause, but constipation with a rectum filled with firm but not hard faeces may also be associated with faecal incontinence.

Once the diagnosis has been made, treatment should be instituted as described in Chapter 14, and then steps taken to ensure that the condition, once treated, does not return. If incontinence remains after constipation has been successfully treated, then a full investigation must be carried out to discover a cause for it within the lower alimentary tract, and there must be a high suspicion of malignant disease.

Symptomatic faecal incontinence

This category includes all those patients with incontinence due to colo-rectal disease, diarrhoea and occasionally other pathologies.

Faecal incontinence in old people may be a presenting symptom of any disorder which produces diarrhoea. It may be that this reflects an age change in the fine control of anal sphincter function in rela-

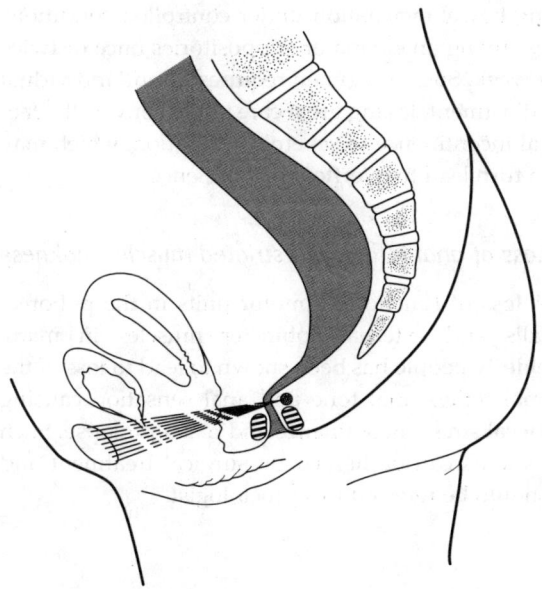

Fig. 9.1 Ano-rectal angle.

tion to a liquid stool, and possibly some impairment of the sampling mechanism of the upper anal canal for distinguishing between liquid faeces and flatus. Diarrhoea is sometimes associated with faecal incontinence in people who are younger. The most common causes of diarrhoea in the elderly are the taking of purgatives and other drugs (for example, iron), carcinoma of the colon or rectum, diverticular disease, distal proctitis, ulcerative colitis, Crohn's disease, ischaemic colitis or gastroenteritis.

All of these indicate the need for proper investigation, including sigmoidoscopy, and it is often necessary to proceed to full colonoscopy, barium enema or barium computed tomogram (CT) examination, depending on the overall clinical picture.

Other occasional causes of symptomatic faecal incontinence are diabetes, thyrotoxicosis, prolapse of the rectum and disruption of the anal sphincter, for example after an incompetent operation for haemorrhoids. The treatment is that of the underlying disorder and if this is untreatable then symptomatic management of faecal incontinence is as that described below for neurogenic incontinence.

Neurogenic faecal incontinence

Loss of cortical inhibition following rectal distention

The normal process of defaecation follows a gastrocolic reflex. This causes movement of a faecal mass from the descending colon into the rectum. This rectal distention is followed by relaxation of the internal sphincter. As in the bladder, no intrinsic rectal contractions occur in the normal adult because central inhibition prevents this.

Generally, if defaecation is not possible, then the act is postponed by the voluntary inhibition of rectal contractions, a rapid return of the contracting tone to the internal sphincter, and contraction of the external sphincter.

In elderly people, however, and particularly in patients suffering from cerebrovascular disease, the ability to postpone the act of defaecation may be impaired or lost. This type of incontinence is seen most characteristically in people who have vascular dementia, other forms of dementia such as Alzheimer's disease, or damage to the cortical inhibitory mechanisms by stroke. The clinical picture is of one or two formed stools found in the bed or clothing each day, and these usually follow meals or hot drinks.

Management of neurogenic faecal incontinence

Management of this condition is to try to prevent the reflex emptying of the colon following rectal distention and to secure bowel motions under controlled conditions. If the incontinent stool is passed after an early morning cup of tea which is given in bed, then the answer is quite simple: the patient should be sat out of the bed comfortably and in privacy on a commode with a blanket around the knees and can be given a cup of tea and remain on the commode until the stool has been passed.

This is no more than good and observant nursing practice, and will be the modus operandi in enlightened hospitals and nursing homes.

If the neurogenic faecal incontinence is not as predictable as this, then it may be controlled by giving a constipating agent such as codeine phosphate or loperamide two or three times a day, and securing bowel evacuation under controlled conditions by giving an enema or suppositories once or twice a week. Such a regimen requires careful individual adjustment, taking great care not to convert the faecal incontinence to severe constipation, which may in turn lead to overflow incontinence.

Loss of anal reflex with striated muscle weakness

A loss of functioning motor units in the puborectalis and external sphincter muscles in many elderly people has been shown to lead to loss of the anal reflex, anal tone and anal sensation causing faecal stress incontinence and rectal prolapse. Such patients can be helped by surgical treatment and should be referred to a proctologist.

Management of environmental factors of faecal incontinence

As is the case with urinary incontinence, a substantial number of patients with faecal incontinence suffer from urgency of defaecation.

In such people the provision of an unobtrusive commode or nearby toilet, or adaptation of clothing so it can be removed easily may drastically reduce or even stop the number of episodes of faecal incontinence. Adaptations to the toilet providing a footstool and grab rail also help frail elderly people with poor mobility to use an ordinary toilet.

Some patients with intractable faecal incontinence which cannot be managed by any of the means mentioned above will need to be supplied with pads and appropriate protective clothing as well as facilities for frequent bathing. Such patients should be very much a minority if faecal incontinence is being assessed and treated properly.

A general approach to the management of faecal incontinence is shown in Figure 9.3. In conclusion, it cannot be overemphasized that persistent faecal incontinence in old people is a failure of medical and nursing practice. It is a matter which must be taken seriously by both doctors and nurses. It is not a normal accompaniment of old age and it may be the first evidence of serious and treatable disease within the bowel or elsewhere.

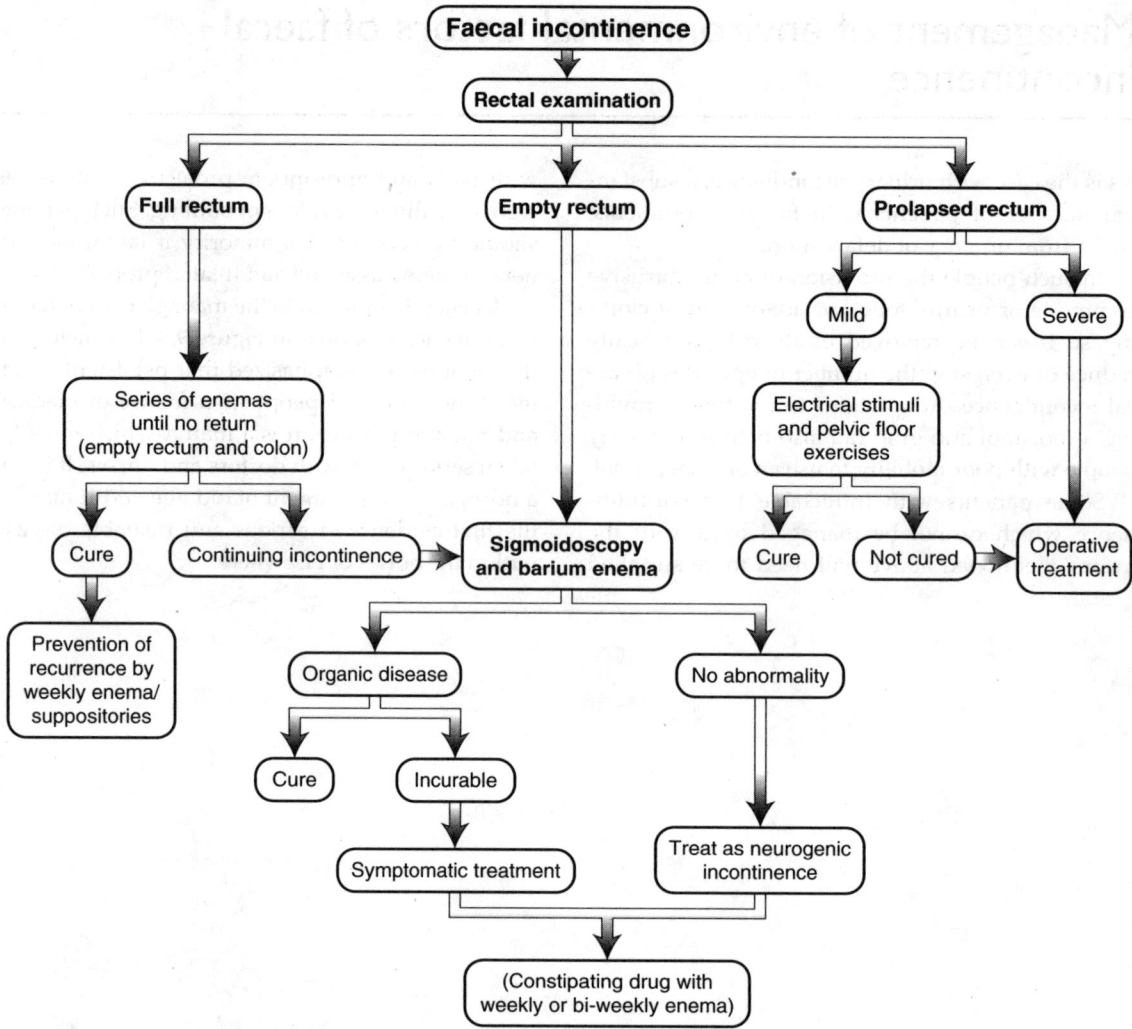

Fig. 9.3 Flow diagram of the diagnosis and management of faecal incontinence.

10

Pressure sores

Introduction

Pressure sores are an important cause of morbidity, and even mortality, in old age. Despite considerable advances in methods of prevention and treatment, pressure sores continue to present a frequent challenge to health care workers. Frail elderly patients are more likely to have clinical problems which predispose to pressure sores so that the incidence tends to increase with age. Of course, a pressure sore can occur in an immobile patient of any age.

What is a pressure sore?

When tissues are deprived of their blood supply by compression or shearing forces for more than about 2 hours necrosis can take place. If pressure is relieved within that time minimal damage takes place and an ulcer does not form. However, when blood flow is not restored, necrosis of the skin and subcutaneous tissues to a variable depth will take place and a pressure sore will form. It is obvious, therefore, that immobility is the most important risk factor.

Patients who are not immobile can lie in bed for many days without developing pressure sores as they can change their position instinctively and frequently to prevent serious tissue ischaemia taking place. Patients unable to make these movements will certainly develop pressure sores unless they are moved by another person or lying on a special pressure-relieving surface.

The pressure required to cause tissue ischaemia is not particularly high. The mean capillary perfusion pressure is about 25 mmHg, so any pressure above that level will stop blood flow and cause necrosis if sustained.

Risk factors

As stated above, immobility is the key risk factor. However, a variety of other factors can also contribute to the overall risk including:

- all conditions which cause severe limitation of mobility including stroke, severe Parkinson's disease, severe bony injury particularly in the lower limbs and pelvis, spinal cord injuries, multiple sclerosis etc.
- any condition causing severe reduction in the level of consciousness, but particularly coma
- any condition causing a reduction in cardiac output or blood pressure, for example cardiogenic shock, septicaemia, gastrointestinal haemorrhage, severe dehydration etc.
- severe underlying arteriosclerotic disease, thereby compromising blood supply to tissues
- certain haematological conditions such as severe anaemia or any cause of hyperviscosity
- severe uncontrolled metabolic conditions such as diabetic ketoacidosis
- sedative or analgesic drugs when these reduce the patient's instinctive and spontaneous movements or reduce the patient's ability to sense pain and discomfort.

This is by no means an exhaustive list but it can be seen that any condition which reduces mobility or the delivery and utilization of oxygen and nutrients to peripheral tissues will predispose to pressure necrosis.

When do pressure sores occur?

Various studies have shown that most episodes of pressure necrosis occur when patients are acutely ill and it is therefore imperative to identify those most at risk and to take preventative action.

Risk charts such as the one shown in Figure 10.1 have been used in both acute and chronic settings to pick out those patients most likely to develop a pressure sore.

However, charts of this type, though helpful, are no substitute for constant vigilance on the part of nursing and medical staff for the individual risk factors outlined above.

PRESSURE SORES – ASSESSMENT OF RISK				
Name of patient: .... Unit no.				
		Date		
	Marks			
General physical condition				
Good	4			
Fair	3			
Poor	2			
Very bad	1			
Mental state				
Alert	4			
Apathetic	3			
Confused	2			
Stuporose	1			
Activity				
Ambulent	4			
Ambulent with help	3			
Chairbound	2			
Confined to bed	1			
Mobility				
Full	4			
Slightly limited	3			
Very limited	2			
Immobile	1			
Incontinence				
Not incontinent	4			
Occasionally incontinent	3			
Usually incontinent of urine	2			
Doubly incontinent	1			
Total				

Fig. 10.1 At risk chart.

Types of mechanical force leading to necrosis

Compression

Direct compression is the commonest and most easily understood mechanical force which causes pressure necrosis. Clearly, the harder the surface a person is lying on, the smaller the area of distribution of weight will be and the higher the pressure will be at the points of contact.

This is clearly illustrated in Figure 10.2. Therefore, pressure at contact points would be very high when the patient is lying on a concrete surface and at its lowest when he or she is floating on a water bed. It is worth remembering that a patient lying flat on an ordinary foam mattress will have tissue pressures of around 60–70 mmHg over the

sacrum and 30–45 mmHg over the heels, which is far in excess of mean capillary perfusion pressure.

As discussed below, many of the special surfaces used in the prevention and treatment of patients with pressure sores are designed to produce pressures at key areas which are below mean capillary perfusion pressure, or which mechanically redistribute the points of compression in cyclical fashion.

Shearing forces

Many bedfast patients do not lie flat but are supported in various semirecumbent positions as shown in Figure 10.3. There is then a tendency for the body to slide forward.

There is a propensity for the skin to adhere to the bedclothes and for the skeleton and musculature to continue to slide under the force of gravity, thereby causing a shearing effect in the subcutaneous tissues.

This can obstruct the small arteries and arterioles by distorting them and thereby compromise the blood supply to subcutaneous tissues and cause necrosis. Of course, patients who are subject to shearing forces are usually simultaneously subjected to compression forces, as shown in Figure 10.3. The skin in the region of the buttocks, the posterior aspect of the legs and the heels is particularly vulnerable to shearing forces, though in certain positions practically any area of skin could be damaged by the same mechanism.

Folding

Movement of the body on a surface which causes adherence of the skin can produce actual folds in the skin itself. This is more likely to happen in emaciated individuals in whom the skin is lax and will only occur in those areas where the skin is not closely tethered to the skeleton.

This is illustrated in Figure 10.4. Folding of the skin will distort and obstruct blood vessels and can thereby lead to ischaemic tissue necrosis. As men-

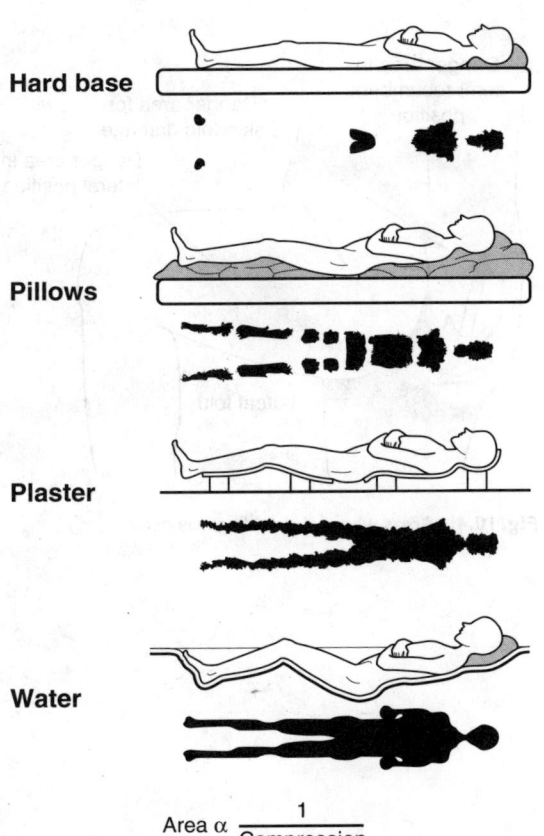

Hard base

Pillows

Plaster

Water

$$\text{Area} \propto \frac{1}{\text{Compression}}$$

Fig. 10.2 Area of the body in contact with various surfaces.

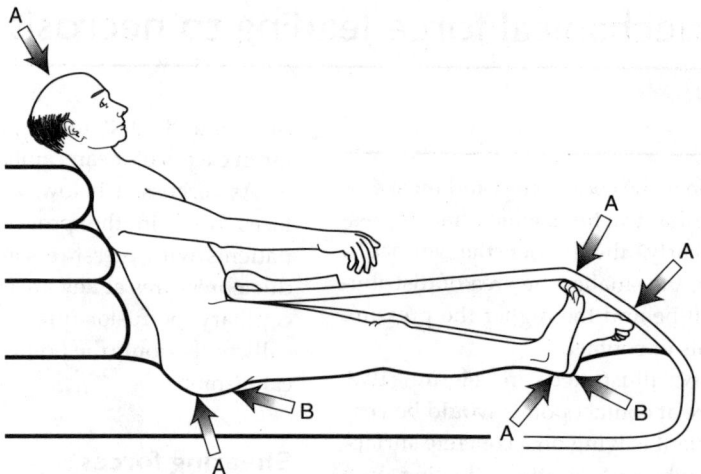

Fig. 10.3 Shearing forces. A = compressing force; B = shearing force. Shearing force depends on friction, which is increased if the bed sheet is wet.

tioned above, patients whose arterial blood supply is already poor as a result of arteriosclerosis will be particularly prone to this type of damage.

Box 10.1 Types of mechanical force leading to necrosis

- Compression causes ischaemia and this will be most apparent when the body is lying on a surface which does not fit its contours.
- Shearing forces cause ischaemia which will be most in evidence when there is a high degree of friction between the body and the surface lain on.
- Folding causes ischaemia and this will be most severe in emaciated individuals.
- Immobility is the basic underlying factor.
- Any mechanical, physiological or metabolic factor which compromises the delivery of oxygen and nutrients to tissue can contribute to the risk of developing a pressure sore.

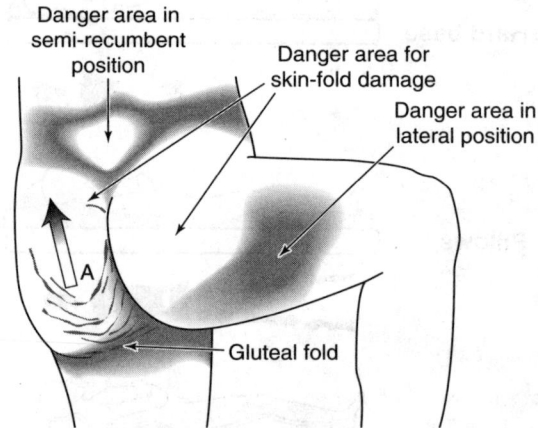

Fig. 10.4 Areas where skin folding may occur.

Prevention

In theory, the prevention of pressure sores is quite simple.

Patients who are at risk should be identified and the compression, shearing and folding effects prevented.

Those with the risk factors listed above are particularly likely to be affected and therefore stand to gain most from preventive measures. Patients identified as at risk should immediately receive special attention including the following:

- whenever possible treatment of all predisposing medical conditions such as hypotension, dehydration, hypoxia, anaemia and sepsis
- turning of the patient every 2 hours by nursing staff or use of special beds such as an alternating pressure mattress, 'low air loss' bed or one of the other many different types of bed designed to reduce compression effects
- additional protection for the heels
- a bed cradle to reduce compression and shearing effects in the feet.

Overcoming immobility

All steps should be taken to improve the patient's general mobility as quickly as possible. In the meantime, pressure necrosis can be avoided by the nursing staff changing the patient's position every 2 hours or thereabouts.

When performed regularly and without fail, this method is very effective but it has a number of limitations including:

1. It is labour-intensive and uses a considerable amount of nursing time.
2. Some patient's medical and surgical conditions prevent it being used either for technical reasons or because of pain.

Under circumstances where regular turning is not appropriate or not possible it is usually necessary to employ a special type of bed. The alternating pressure mattress is a tried and tested method which is successful when used properly. The principles of this are illustrated in Figure 10.5.

There are various models of this type of mattress on the market and most have inflatable cells of about 12 cm (5 inches) diameter and a pump cycle of 7–10 minutes.

The main disadvantages are:

1. mechanical failure which can go unnoticed
2. inadvertent switching off of the pump.

In either of these cases the patient is particularly at risk from pressure necrosis as nursing staff may assume that the device is working and therefore not turn the patient or check that all is well.

Other ways of diminishing compression forces

One of the most useful and versatile appliances for nursing very immobile patients is the 'low air loss bed'. This consists of a number of large cells each with its own pressure control system. Therefore, the pressure in each cell can be adjusted, once the patient is in place, to a pressure which is below mean capillary perfusion pressure. Furthermore, the constant leak of a small amount of warm air from the surface of the cells helps to keep the skin dry and to prevent maceration. The main principles

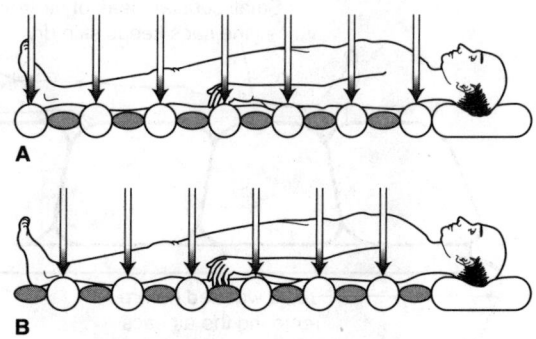

- Inflate before patient goes on it
- Watch for failure
- Patient to be as recumbent as possible

Fig. 10.5 Alternating pressure mattress.

of the low air loss bed are illustrated in Figure 10.6.

A number of water beds are also available which allow the patient to lie with about half the body surface immersed in water. The water is in a fabric envelope contained within a rigid trough and sufficiently voluminous to hold the half-submerged body.

There is a heating element to keep the water at a suitable temperature. The main difficulty with the water bed is nursing the patient, and this method is not suitable for those who are incontinent. It is also very difficult for patients to get in and out of the water bed and may, therefore, tend to increase the period of bedfastness. Water beds which stand on adjustable-height hospital beds tend to make the patients easier to nurse. Some patients with severe painful joint conditions are probably best nursed on a water bed and in these circumstances the method can be very successful.

Preventing shearing forces

Shearing forces can be prevented either by sitting patients out of bed or lying them flat in bed. The risk is also increased when patients lie in wet beds, thereby increasing the coefficient of friction. If the patient has to be nursed in the erect sitting position, then it may be helpful to arrange the bed with a board at the foot to prevent sliding forward. Care should always be taken to protect the feet of elderly patients from the pressure of the bedclothing; the bed should not be made too tightly, and the use of a bed cradle should be considered. There are various makes of mattress cover available to help reduce shearing forces and the use of these should be considered in individual patients. Furthermore, a properly adjusted low air loss bed can also be used to sit patients up without causing too much shearing.

Preventing folding of the skin

Most of the precautions mentioned under the prevention of shearing will also help to prevent folding of the skin. Nursing staff should pay particular attention to the positioning of patients, particularly when they are emaciated, so as not to leave tight skin folds in place for prolonged periods of time.

When any of the preventive measures above are being applied it is vital that nursing and medical staff inspect the patient's skin, particularly over vulnerable areas such as the sacrum, to detect the early signs of damage due to pressure, shearing or folding. When very minimal damage has occurred there will simply be transient erythema and if action is taken at this time necrosis and ulceration can be avoided.

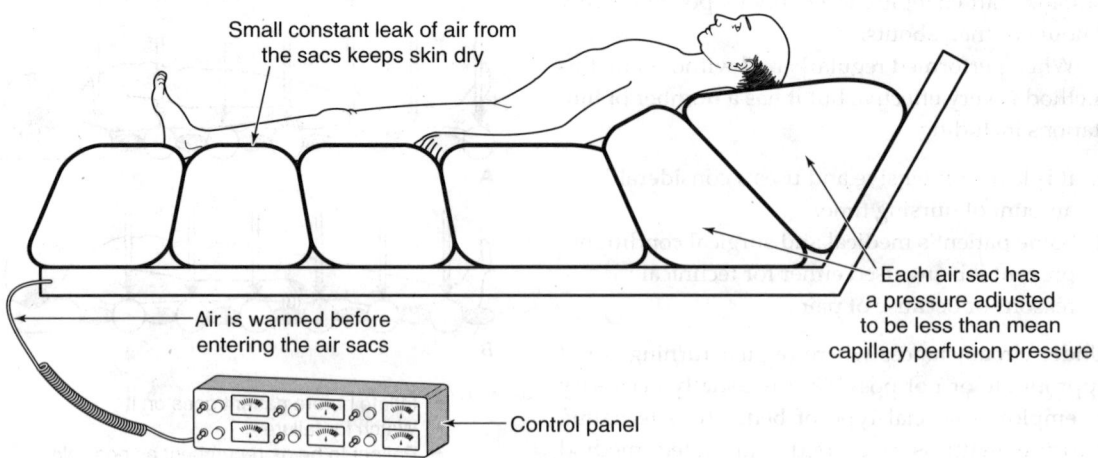

Small constant leak of air from the sacs keeps skin dry

Air is warmed before entering the air sacs

Each air sac has a pressure adjusted to be less than mean capillary perfusion pressure

Control panel

Fig. 10.6 The low air loss bed.

Special precautions for the prevention of sores on the heels

Pressure sores on the heels deserve a special mention because they are common, often take a long time to heal if the blood supply to the lower limbs is poor, and can result in a considerable delay in mobilizing the patient if they cause pain on standing.

A variety of methods can be used to help distribute the weight and thereby reduce compression on the heels. These include some of the special types of bed mentioned above and also specially contoured foam pads to rest the heels on in bed, thereby reducing pressure, friction and shearing forces. Care must be taken not to cause any obstruction to venous return as this will predispose to deep venous thrombosis. The careful use of pillows around the lower limbs can be part of the routine nursing care of very immobile patients and will also help to reduce compression if the pillows are positioned to support the whole of the lower limb including the heels, with frequent changes of position and review of the vulnerable areas.

The treatment of established pressure sores

The methods discussed above for the prevention of pressure sores should, of course, be instigated at once if a pressure sore is present and, if it is severe or the patient is very immobile, the use of one of the special types of bed should be considered.

At this stage pressure sores are often graded according to severity (see Box 10.2).

Box 10.2 Severity of pressure sores

- *Grade 1* An area of erythema without necrosis or ulceration. These sores simply require immediate institution of preventative measures to prevent any further progression to a more severe grade.
- *Grade 2* Ulceration of the skin with little necrosis of subcutaneous tissues and no involvement of underlying muscles or other structures.
- *Grade 3* A deeper ulcer with necrosis of deep structures including muscle.
- *Grade 4* A very severe ulcer with exposure of deep structures such as bone and tendons and the formation of extensive undermining cavities.

It is important to control infection, particularly if there is cellulitis in the surrounding healthy tissue.

If the patient is febrile or has a leucocytosis it is important to act quickly to control the infection.

Local cleansing of the tissue will control minor degrees of infection, though systemic antibiotics will usually be required if the patient has cellulitis or is bacteraemic. Complete sterility of the ulcer is not possible, or necessary for the healing process.

Black eschars and necrotic tissue must be removed before healing can take place properly. Removal of necrotic tissue sometimes requires minor surgical procedures and the use of proteolytic enzyme solutions. Enzymes can be introduced directly in powder form or injected into deep necrotic tissue. The most widely used preparation is a mixture of streptokinase and streptodornase. The complete removal of necrotic tissue often takes many days of patient trimming and re-dressing.

Once the sore is clean and free of eschar and necrotic tissue, healing will proceed naturally at a rate dependent on a number of factors including:

1. *The blood supply to the tissues in the region of the ulcer.* If blood supply is normal, healing will proceed quite quickly with the development of granulation tissue. In such patients there is a temperature difference of about 2.5°C between the area of the sore and the area of the surrounding skin.

On the other hand, when the blood supply is poor as in patients with severe arteriosclerosis, the temperature difference is much lower, usually less than 1°C, and healing is very slow or may not proceed at all.

2. *The patient's nutritional status.* Patients who are well nourished from the point of view of protein, energy and vitamin C will have the optimal rate of healing of their pressure sore.

3. *Whether patients suffer from certain conditions.* Healing will be delayed in patients with a low cardiac output, anaemia, underlying malignant disease, or uncontrolled metabolic conditions such as hyperglycaemia, chronic renal failure, and sepsis etc.

In some patients the healing needs to be augmented by plastic surgery, either in the form of closure of large ulcer craters or skin grafting.

It should be noted that the continued use of oxidizing cleansing agents such as Eusol after the sore has been cleared of necrotic fragments can damage granulation tissue and thereby actually delay healing.

Therefore, it can be seen that the principles of treatment are based on:

- relief and avoidance of compression, shearing and folding
- cleaning and debriding the sore and controlling infection
- improving the patient's general condition and nutritional status as much as possible. Patients with moderate or severe anaemia should receive a blood transfusion and/or haematinic treatment to raise their haemoglobin.

There are a vast number of dressings and appliances available for the treatment of pressure sores. The evidence that any one of these is superior to the others is not particularly strong. However, those which help to redistribute pressure, help to keep the sore clean, and do not inhibit the growth of granulation tissue or epithelium are suitable. There is no evidence that anabolic steroids or hyperoxygenation are of any benefit.

After healing has been achieved all measures must be taken to reduce immobility and prevent further ulceration taking place.

Bone disease and fractures

Introduction

Whilst a wide range of bone conditions, including various tumours, can be encountered in old age, there are three kinds of bone disease which are common in old people; these are osteoporosis, osteomalacia and Paget's disease (osteitis deformans). All three give rise to bone pain and predispose to fractures, but they are very different in their underlying pathophysiology. The first two are disorders of bone metabolism, and therefore generalized, though with local variations in intensity. On the other hand, Paget's disease is a localized or multifocal but never generalized disease, the pathogenesis and aetiology of which has come to be understood a little better in recent years.

Osteoporosis

Osteoporosis is numerically the most important metabolic bone condition in Europe and North America and certain other parts of the world.

It is particularly prevalent amongst postmenopausal white women, though under certain circumstances and in the presence of certain predisposing factors the condition can be seen in men or women of any race.

A huge amount of research has been performed to try to obtain an understanding of the aetiology and pathogenesis of osteoporosis, but no single common factor has been identified other than that the subjects must have been in negative calcium balance for a substantial length of time. Nevertheless, the following points can be made with some confidence:

- The fundamental change is reduction in the total amount of bone in the skeleton.
- The microscopic appearance and structural histology of affected bone is normal.
- Chemical analysis of bone after ashing reveals no significant change in the proportions of bone-forming elements, though it is acknowledged that this is a fairly crude method of analysing chemical content which would not reveal possible changes of molecular structure.
- The serum calcium and phosphate concentrations and the serum alkaline phosphatase level are within normal limits.

Normal bone content of the skeleton

Measurements of the total amount of bone at various ages in a large cross-section of the population have shown an increase up to the age of around 30; the total bone content then remains approximately constant till about the age of 45, after which it falls progressively in both sexes, but more rapidly after the menopause in women. It might be argued, therefore, that osteroporosis is a physiological effect of advancing age, and that clinical osteroporosis only emerges when total bone is reduced below some critical level at which fractures are more likely to occur. Indeed, there is some evidence that those who have an above-average amount of bone at maturity will lose it in the same way as their less well-endowed cohorts, but in old age they can still be left with enough bone to bear the body weight and to resist the breaking forces of muscle action without developing fractures.

Risk factors for osteoporosis

Epidemiological and clinical evidence gathered over the last 15 years or so has given us a substantial understanding of those factors which are associated with an increased risk of developing clinically important osteoporosis.

It must be stressed that many of these factors are at play for many decades, or even throughout the patient's life, and only manifest as clinical osteoporosis in old age. It is obvious, therefore, that any strategies aimed at reducing the prevalence of osteoporosis must take this prolonged time span into account. The most important risk factors for osteoporosis are outlined in Box 11.1.

Box 11.1 Risk factors for osteoporosis

- Strong family history
- Prolonged immobility
- House-bound and not exposed to direct sunlight
- Poor calcium intake
- Smoking
- Heavy alcohol intake
- Malabsorption and malnutrition
- Postmenopausal, particularly with premature menopause
- Any cause of prolonged amenorrhoea
- Long-term high-dose corticosteroid therapy
- Thyrotoxicosis
- Hyperparathyroidism
- Hypogonadism
- Anorexia nervosa

It can be seen from the box that some of these causes are inevitable and cannot be avoided, such as strong family history or the menopause. However, other predisposing risk factors are amenable to treatment, such as causes of oestrogen deficiency (including the menopause), or can be avoided altogether, such as cigarette smoking.

Once people reach old age the same risk factors still apply but it is particularly important in elderly patients to ensure that there is not a prolonged period of unnecessary immobility, unnecessary treatment with corticosteroid drugs and a diet with sufficient calcium and vitamin D to minimize the rate at which bone loss is occurring.

Clinical features of osteoporosis

Osteoporosis is not in itself a symptomatic condition, and it can exist for many years without the patient being aware of it. However, when bone fracture starts to occur, including small incremental fracturing of the spine, pain is the main symptom. Clinically, the spine appears to be affected earliest and worst.

Therefore, backache is an important common and early symptom of osteoporosis and is usually felt in the lower dorsal or lumbar regions.

It is often relieved by lying flat and made worse by twisting movements of the trunk. Girdle pain from nerve root compression occurs rarely, though some patients do present with sciatic nerve compression. The symptoms are often curiously intermittent, with sudden exacerbations of pain being followed by months of freedom from discomfort, without any obvious corresponding changes in the appearance on ordinary radiographs.

Crush fractures of one dorsal or lumbar vertebra or more are a frequent finding in osteoporosis, though there is a fairly weak relationship between the extent of these fractures and the patient's complaints of pain. The manner in which crush fracture and vertebral body compression alter the length and shape of the spine is indicated in Figure 11.1. The objective physical signs of osteoporosis are unimpressive. A dorsal kyphosis is common and there is not usually much scoliosis. The back is usually smoothly rounded unless angulated by the wedging effect of a crush fracture. Loss of height and downward inclination of the head are two byproducts of severe crush fractures.

Osteoporosis also predisposes to the fracture of other bones. The neck of the femur, pubic rami, the forearm and upper end of the humerus are particularly liable to fracture in patients with osteoporosis. Thus the physical appearance of a patient with osteoporosis is summarized in Figure 11.2.

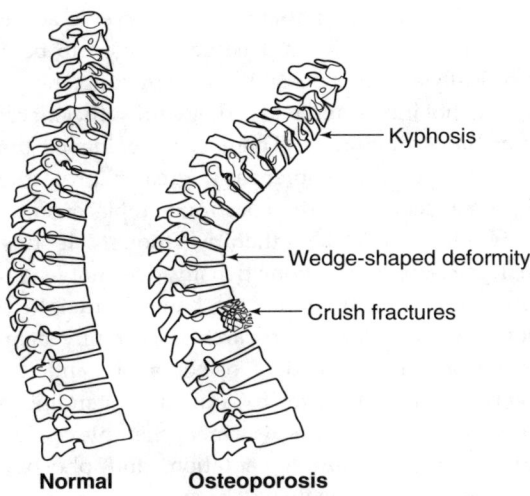

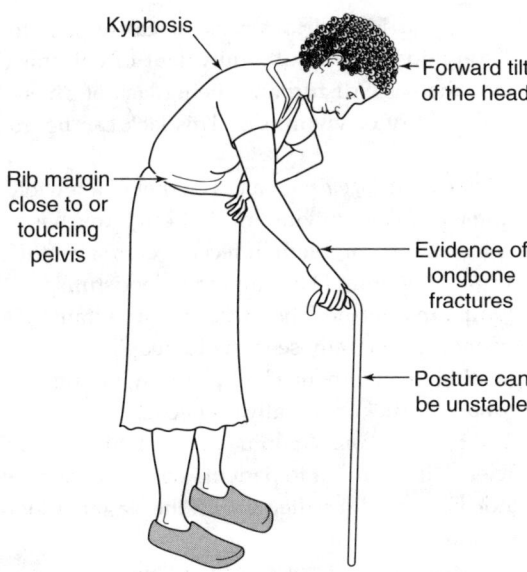

Normal　　**Osteoporosis**

Fig. 11.1　In osteoporosis the spine becomes shortened and more curved (kyphosis).

Fig. 11.2　The typical appearance of a patient with advanced osteoporosis.

Investigations

Radiological findings. On plain radiographs, loss of radiological density in the vertebral bodies is the main finding, though standardization of bone density by this method is difficult. Crush fractures seen on lateral radiographs of the spine in a patient with severe generalized osteopenia is most likely to be due to osteoporosis, though care must be taken not to miss other pathology such as myeloma or metastatic malignancy. Paucity of trabecular marking is a more reliable radiological feature of osteoporosis of the femoral head and neck, and the Singh index, which is based on femoral head and neck trabecular markings, correlates reasonably well with post-mortem chemical analysis of bone. Bone density can be measured more accurately using dual energy X-ray absorption (dexa) analysis.

This method is of some use in the diagnosis of osteoporosis in difficult cases, but is more useful in tracking the rate of change in individuals before and after treatment. There is reasonable, but not perfect, correlation between the results of dexa scanning and post-mortem measurement of the tensile strength of bone.

Blood tests. There is no diagnostic blood test for osteoporosis, and as already mentioned, the serum calcium, phosphate and alkaline phosphatase levels are normal. However, blood tests can be used to identify some of the risk factors such as severe oestrogen deficiency, other forms of hypogonadism, thyrotoxicosis and various deficiency states.

Treatment of established osteoporosis

A number of treatments have now been shown to decrease the rate of bone loss, decrease the risk of certain types of fracture, and in some cases improve mineralization of bone. Thus, in an elderly female patient with radiological changes suggestive of osteoporosis in whom a fracture has occurred, the treatments outlined in Box 11.2 would be appropriate. Of course, concomitant disease must be taken into account and the final decision as to whether or not to go ahead with these treatments must depend on the physician's judgement as to whether the patient is likely to gain overall benefit.

Box 11.2 Drug treatment of established osteoporosis

- Patients with established vertebral disease can benefit from cyclical treatment with etidronate and calcium.
- There is evidence that calcium and vitamin D supplementation reduces the rate of a second fracture in elderly postmenopausal women.
- Hormone replacement therapy (HRT) should be considered, particularly in women with established osteoporosis in the immediate postmenopausal or perimenopausal phase.

Prophylaxis in patients at risk of osteoporosis

Clearly, all those modifiable risk factors outlined in Box 11.1 should be dealt with as far as possible and preferably while the patient is still young and does not have clinical osteoporosis. Some patients obviously fall into very high risk groups and these can be summarized as below:

The following patients should almost invariably receive oestrogen replacement therapy:

- patients with early menopause (menopause at 45 or younger)
- patients requiring long-term use of corticosteriods
- patients with a prolonged history of anorexia nervosa
- patients with a history of late menarche (15 years of age or older)
- patients with secondary amenorrhoea
- those with chronic liver disease
- those with a history of prolonged bed rest.

The patients in the following categories should also be considered for oestrogen replacement therapy, though the evidence of benefit is less clear-cut:

- osteoporosis in a primary relative
- heavy smokers
- heavy drinkers
- women who are very concerned about osteoporosis and have asked to receive oestrogen replacement therapy.

Of course, all such patients should receive advice on lifestyle and diet and be encouraged to be as physically active as possible, stop smoking, moderate alcohol intake and take a diet with sufficient calcium and vitamin D. There is no evidence that anabolic steroids confer any greater protection against osteoporosis than oestrogen replacement.

Similarly, fluoride therapy, though it does increase radiological bone density, does not lead to any improvement in the mechanical strength of bone. A great deal of research is currently being performed in the field of osteoporosis, and it is likely that as time goes by, our understanding of how to use hormone replacement therapy, calcium and vitamin D supplementation, and phosphonates such as etidronate will become more sophisticated and our ability to modify the progress of osteoporosis will improve.

Osteomalacia

Osteomalacia is due to a lack of calcium in the skeleton and is the adult equivalent of childhood rickets, the basic disturbance being lack of physiological activity of vitamin D. This lack can be due to:

1. *Simple dietary deficiency.* The diet of a few old people is deficient in vitamin D, though this has become less of a problem in recent years since the addition of vitamin D to numerous foodstuffs, including margarine. Therefore, dietary vitamin D deficiency is generally seen in old people who are neglecting to feed themselves properly, taking a very narrow diet or actually cachectic.

2. *Malabsorption.* Vitamin D is fat-soluble, so a deficiency is common in patients with any cause of steatorrhoea and in patients with the stagnant loop syndrome.

3. *Inadequate skin exposure to sunlight.* The ultraviolet component of sunlight is needed for vitamin D synthesis. In countries such as the United Kingdom, other parts of northern Europe and some parts of North America, the relative lack of sunlight and prolonged cold winters result in very few elderly patients exposing substantial skin areas to sunlight for many months of the year. Of course, in countries with a warm sunny climate, such as Australia, this will be much less of a

problem. Particularly vulnerable are frail, house-bound patients, and patients with deeply pigmented skins living in countries with relatively little direct sunlight, particularly when the dietary intake of vitamin D is only marginally adequate.

Therefore, an example of a group particularly at risk would be elderly Asian women living in the North of England.

Clinical features of osteomalacia

Often the diagnosis of osteomalacia is made simply by keeping the possibility in mind when the patient's circumstances predispose to the disease. There are no particularly typical symptoms or signs, though the following should be looked for:

- generalized muscle pains, especially backache
- muscular weakness and stiffness
- tenderness of the bones to pressure
- pathological fracture with no evidence of malignancy
- skeletal deformity.

Generalized muscle pains are common but are sometimes misdiagnosed as being due to arthritis or polymyalgia rheumatica. Examination will, however, often reveal striking muscle weakness which is due to a specific myopathy, and is associated with changes in the electromyogram. The weakness affects the proximal limb girdle muscles.

Flexors of the hip are worst affected and make it difficult to lift the foot clear of the ground. This difficulty is avoided in some patients by adopting a stumpy waddling gait.

In the shoulder, much more rarely involved, abduction and elevation of the arm are weak and interfere with dressing and hair toilet.

The bones are softened as a result of the lack of calcium and this has three effects:

- There is pain on weight-bearing.
- The bones are tender to pressure, the ribs and sternum are most accessible for this sign.
- The bones fracture easily.

Confirming the diagnosis of osteomalacia

On plain radiographs the bones are less dense than normal. Most often affected are the vertebral bod-ies, the upper and lower surfaces of which become concave. Crush fractures are not typical of osteomalacia, but osteoporosis coexists frequently, in which case crush fractures may also be present.

One sign which is pathognomonic, though not always present, is Looser's zones. These resemble crack fractures; they are perpendicular to the external bone surface and reach to it, with denser ridges of apparent callus on either side. The ribs, scapula, neck of the humerus and femoral neck are common sites for Looser's zones.

There are usually serum biochemical abnormalities in osteomalacia, in contrast with osteoporosis. The serum calcium concentration is low and reverts to normal when vitamin D treatment is given.

In elderly patients the serum phosphate level is not reliable in the diagnosis of osteomalacia. Most patients, however, will have a raised alkaline phosphatase. Bone biopsy is not routinely necessary for making the diagnosis, though it is sometimes performed during surgery for fracture in a patient with osteomalacia. Histological examination of a section of such a biopsy, without decalcification, will show the typical increase in the volume and thickness of osteoid and a decrease in the staining intensity of the calcification front.

Treatment of osteomalacia

There are two essential elements of treatment. These are:

- treatment with vitamin D
- removal of any conditions which predispose to vitamin D deficiency wherever possible.

Oral calciferol treatment is often sufficient, though some clinicians recommend an initial intramuscular dose of 50 000 units of vitamin D to be given and then followed by oral therapy.

Patients with severe renal failure are unable to convert calciferol to the active form of vitamin D and should therefore receive 1-alpha hydroxycholecalciferol.

Calcium supplements should be given simultaneously to provide calcium for incorporation in bone and to avoid a sudden fall in serum calcium concentration. Some patients with major predisposition to vitamin D deficiency, such as house-bound elderly patients, should receive a regular vitamin D supplement to avoid a relapse of osteomalacia.

Vitamin D therapy is not entirely without risk. Excessive dosage can rapidly cause hypercalcaemia, with the attendant risk of calcifying soft tissues or organs. It is, therefore, wise to keep the patient under observation and to control calciferol dosage according to the serum calcium concentration. Very rarely, the patient will become habituated to vitamin D for its euphorizing effect.

Paget's disease of bone

Paget's disease of bone is a patchy disease of the skeleton. Any bone can be affected but there seems to be a predilection for involvement of the axial skeleton and the long bones are also frequently involved.

In the affected area there is simultaneous reabsorption of bone and the formation of new bone, but this new bone has a disordered architectural pattern and is of reduced tensile strength. Consequently, it is more liable to fracture under stress.

In some parts of the world it is relatively common, including the United Kingdom, other parts of northern Europe and parts of North America, with intermediate levels of prevalence in South Africa and Australasia and very low incidence in Southeast Asia and Japan.

In those areas where the prevalence is high, the disease is seen in people of all races and ethnic backgrounds. As a large proportion of Paget's disease is asymptomatic the true overall prevalence is unknown, though it is estimated to be between 1% and 2% of the total population in the United Kingdom.

The aetiology of Paget's disease

The cause of Paget's disease of bone is not known for certain. However, recent research has shown inclusion bodies in pagetic osteoclasts which have many of the morphological features of paramyxoviruses, particularly canine distemper virus. There also seems to be a higher prevalence of the disease in countries where people live in close proximity to dogs. While this does not prove that the disease has a viral aetiology it is fairly strong circumstantial evidence.

The clinical features of Paget's disease

These obviously vary according to which bones are affected and how advanced the disease is. The following points should be borne in mind:

- Most Paget's disease is probably asymptomatic.
- The most important symptoms of Paget's disease are pain and bone deformity.
- Patients who have Paget's disease of the skull may complain of deafness if the ossicles are involved or the 8th nerve is compressed at the level of the 8th nerve foramen.
- In active Paget's disease the pagetic bone may feel warmer than surrounding bone and is often tender on compression.

Important complications of Paget's disease

Pathological fracture through pagetic bone is the most common complication. Operative fixation is often necessary, though in a large proportion of cases the patient is left with an ununited fracture.

Osteogenic sarcoma occurs in a small percentage (probably about 1–2%) of pagetic bones. It grows rapidly, metastasizes early and has a poor prognosis unless treated at an early stage. High-output cardiac failure will only occur with very severe wide spread Paget's disease and is very rare. It must be remembered that when heart failure occurs in a patient with Paget's disease it is usually due to one of the common causes of heart disease and not Paget's disease itself.

Investigations of Paget's disease

Plain radiographs of a pagetic bone will show characteristic changes including a prominent resorption front when the disease is active, replacement of normal bone with bone of disordered architecture, and deformity of the shape of the bone. The disease process usually stops at joint surfaces.

The serum calcium and phosphate levels are normal, although the alkaline phosphatase level will be high in a patient with active Paget's disease. Urine hydroxyproline secretion is also markedly increased, though this test is not usually necessary for the routine clinical management of the patient.

Treatment of Paget's disease

Asymptomatic Paget's disease requires no treatment, and analgesics such as paracetamol are often sufficient to control mild to moderate bone pain.

Patients with more severe pain should receive biphosphonate therapy. This is probably best given by using intravenous pamidronate, 30 mg weekly for 6 consecutive weeks. The mode of action is by inhibition of osteoclast activity and by altering calcium appatite crystals in such a way as to slow down bone reabsorption.

Human calcitonin can also be used to suppress bone reabsorption and control pain in Paget's disease, though its cost and the potential complications of treatment have led to it taking second place to biphosphonate therapy for Paget's disease. There is some evidence that control of the pagetic process with biphosphonates can modify the final degree of bone deformity and this may be of particular importance in patients with disfiguring Paget's disease of the facial bones.

Fractures

Introduction

The subject of bone fractures is obviously a very large one and the student is referred to major textbooks for detailed reading.

However, in elderly patients one extremely important site of bone fracture is the upper end of the femur. Women are affected three times more than men and osteoporosis, again much commoner in the female sex, is a major predisposing factor. Fracture of the femoral neck is always a major event, and often a catastrophe which transforms life for the worse in an old person. The main sites of fracture are outlined in Figure 11.3.

Generally speaking, patients with subcapital and transcervical fractures have a relatively low immediate mortality whereas those with intertrochanteric and subtrochanteric fractures (about 40% of the total) tend to be rather older and have a higher immediate mortality.

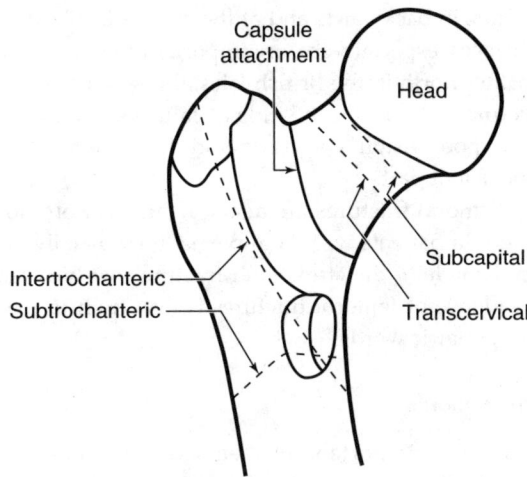

Fig. 11.3 Diagram of various types of fracture of the neck of the femur.

Causes

Fractures in young people usually require severe direct trauma, but in old people they often occur without external violence. The vast majority are in fact due to falls occurring in the home. Direct impact of the fractured area against the ground is probably only one factor. Normally, the main breaking stress on bones comes from the powerful forces exerted by muscles inserted into them, and body weight plays only a minor part. Old people have reduced postural sense and poor righting reflexes compared with the young. Consequently, they trip or stumble easily and recover clumsily, and incoordinated muscle contractions in attempting to recover balance probably have a part to play in femoral neck fractures. About three-quarters of all femoral fractures occur in the home or near it, the commonest place being the dining or sitting room, followed by the kitchen and bedroom. Surprisingly, the bathroom or lavatory is an unusual venue for a fall. Tripping or stumbling over flooring materials is by far the single commonest cause; a ruck in a carpet or a slippery mat are frequently responsible. Falls from a chair or bed, drop attacks, postural hypotension with fainting and giddiness due to vestibular abnormalities are also common circumstances.

Falls outside the home occur on irregular pavements, in back yards and at the curb side. Slippery surfaces, especially ice, are important in winter; the farther north in the British Isles, the larger the part ice plays. In all these kinds of fall, poor illumination, poor vision, confusion and distraction play a consistent part.

Femoral fractures are also a relatively common event in patients with hemiplegia; they usually fall to the side of the stroke and fracture that hip. The incidence of femoral fractures is also high in psychogeriatric wards.

Prevention

The most important elements of prevention of femoral fracture can be summarized as follows:

- reducing the severity of osteoporosis by the measures outlined earlier in this chapter
- reducing environmental hazards within the patient's home as much as possible
- treating medical conditions which might predispose to falling, such as postural hypotension
- avoiding whenever possible drug therapy which might predispose to falls, such as long-acting hypnotics and drugs which cause postural hypotension
- in patients who fall frequently, reducing the risk of hip fracture by the wearing of padded hip protectors.

Treatment

Immediate treatment. Extensive studies have shown that old people with fractured hips have a better outcome if they are treated in a trauma centre in the first instance. This enables them to have rapid assessment of the trauma, to be stabilized haemodynamically and to have any concurrent medical conditions brought under optimal control before operative fixation of the fracture. Once the patients are in optimal condition the fracture should be treated surgically without further delay.

The exact choice of surgical fixation will depend on the site of the fracture. The patient should be operated upon by the most experienced clinician available and attention should be paid intra-operatively and postoperatively to the prevention of pressure sores, infection, deep venous thrombosis and pulmonary embolism.

In a small minority of patients, surgical measures are not undertaken because of the patient's poor general condition or due to the presence of a specific contraindication such as disseminated malignancy.

Orthogeriatric rehabilitation. Once the patient has recovered from the immediate effects of surgery, rehabilitation should begin with the primary aim of enabling the patient to become mobile as soon as possible. Because femoral neck fracture is so common and because early intensive rehabilitation has been shown to be effective, many hospitals, particularly in the United Kingdom, have created specialized orthogeriatric rehabilitation units to take over the patient's care at this stage.

The main aims of orthogeriatric rehabilitation can be summarized as follows:

- to mobilize the patient as soon as possible
- to obtain good pain control with minimum side-effects during the process of rehabilitation
- to investigate the patient when necessary for the cause of falls and to correct any treatable causes, e.g. blackouts due to a rhythm disorder or postural hypotension
- to use the full range of rehabilitation techniques, including physiotherapy and occupational therapy, to enable the patient to achieve as good a level of independence as possible prior to discharge
- to plan discharge from hospital carefully, to organize any additional services required, and to help the patient reduce the risk of environmental hazards which might cause further falls at home
- to bring any other concurrent medical problems under optimum control while the patient is in the orthogeriatric unit and investigate further if necessary; the patient's nutritional status can be reviewed and adjusted when necessary.

Part 3

Special features of disease in old age

12

Anaemia

Introduction

Anaemia may be seen as a consequence of many of the common disease processes encountered in old age and is therefore an important and common problem in geriatric medicine. One widely used definition of anaemia in old age is the World Health Organization criterion of a peripheral blood haemoglobin (Hb) concentration below 130 gm/1 in men and below 120 gm/1 in women. There are a large number of specific causes of anaemia, a full account of which is outside the scope of this book, though some of the more common causes of anaemia in old people are outlined in Box 12.1.

Box 12.1 Some important causes of anaemia in old people

- Iron deficiency (see text)
- Vitamin B$_{12}$ and folate deficiencies (see text)
- The anaemia of chronic diseases (see text)
- Chronic renal failure
- Myelodysplasia
- Malignant infiltration of bone marrow
- Leukaemia
- Hypothyroidism

For the purpose of this chapter, and to illustrate the approach to the investigation and management of anaemia in old people, we will look in some detail at three of the most important reasons for anaemia in old people, which are as follows:

- iron deficiency
- megaloblastic anaemias
- anaemia associated with chronic diseases.

The effects of ageing on the blood

Ageing in the haemopoietic system is an aspect of gerontology where our understanding is very incomplete. The pattern of development of red and white cells is not qualitatively changed as age advances, but the peripheral marrow contains substantially fewer haemopoietic cells and its capacity to respond to artificial stimuli, such as certain polysaccharides and corticosteroids, is reduced. The regenerative response to blood loss or to treatment of pernicious anaemia is also less brisk in old people. On the other hand, the lifespan of red cells is not changed as age advances and their morphology shows no important alteration.

Symptoms and signs of anaemia in elderly people

Patients may complain of a variety of symptoms, some of which are due to the anaemia itself and some to the underlying pathology.

Symptoms

Old people experience much the same symptoms of anaemia as do younger patients. These include:

- easy fatigue
- dyspnoea and palpitations on exertion
- dizziness and lightheadedness
- nonspecific symptoms such as headache,

irritability, failure of concentration and coldness of the limbs

- in elderly patients, declining mobility, falls, confusion or incontinence
- symptoms of vascular insufficiency which may be worsened by anaemia, such as angina or intermittent claudication.

Signs

There may be very few physical signs, though pallor is often present. It can be detected in the face, palms of the hands, soles of the feet and mucous membranes of the lips or conjunctivae; each of these sites can at times be misleading taken individually, but together they provide a reliable guide to anaemia.

Other signs of value are:

- *dystrophic nail changes*. Full-blown koilonychia is almost pathognomonic of iron deficiency but lesser changes such as brittleness, flattening and ridging of the nails are common in the absence of anaemia and are of little diagnostic value.
- *glossitis*. The tongue is reddened, sore and smooth because the papillae are shrunken and flat. These changes occur in many patients with pernicious anaemia and in a few with iron deficiency.

Some other signs, which are not specific but can be due to anaemia, include:

- ankle oedema
- low-grade fever
- weight loss.

Special features of anaemia in the elderly

There are no features of anaemia which are absolutely unique to elderly patients but the following points should be borne in mind.

- The anaemia is sometimes very severe by the time the patient seeks advice; this is probably due mainly to misguided acceptance of symptoms as one of the inevitable evils of getting old, in part to reluctance to bother the

medical attendant, and in part to adjustments in the oxygen dissociation curve.

- Congestive heart failure is a common presenting feature, no doubt because the patient often has intrinsic heart disease as well, and the stage is already set for the development of heart failure.
- Mental symptoms are common and may dominate the scene. Here again, anaemia may be simply the final factor tipping the balance in a patient with failing mental powers.

Iron deficiency anaemia

Iron deficiency is by far the commonest kind of anaemia in old people and is of special importance because it is often the presenting feature of some major disease.

The three basic mechanisms of iron deficiency are:

- blood loss
- malabsorption
- malnutrition.

Iron balance

Iron deficiency anaemia arises when the amount of iron present and available in the marrow falls below that needed for haemoglobin synthesis in developing red cells. This will only arise after the main body iron stores, chiefly in the liver, have already been heavily drained. These reserves are large, about 1000 mg, and are kept constant through a sensitive feedback mechanism in intestinal epithelial cells, which adjust the amount of iron absorbed from the diet to the amount lost to the environment.

The daily iron loss is about 1 mg in healthy individuals, chiefly as exfoliated intestinal cells, plus a small leakage of blood. With a normal iron intake, there is only a small margin available for adjusting to increased losses.

In Europe and North America the dietary iron of old people is in the 8–12 mg range per day, but only about 3–5 mg of this can be absorbed even when absorption is stretched to full capacity. If blood loss exceeds 15 ml per day (7 mg of elemental iron) and even if absorption is increased to the maximum possible, iron stores will decline and iron deficiency anaemia will eventually appear.

The peripheral blood in iron deficiency anaemia

The typical changes in iron deficiency anaemia, in addition to the obvious reduction in haemoglobin concentration, are as follows:

- The mean corpuscular volume (MCV) is reduced below 80 cubic micrometers, and will typically be in the 65–70 cubic micrometer range in a moderately severe case.
- The mean total corpuscular Hb (MCH) is consistently reduced below 30 picograms.
- The peripheral blood film reveals red cells smaller than normal on average, in keeping with the low MCV, but there is a wide range of sizes (anisocytosis) and of shapes (poikilocytosis).

Investigation of iron deficiency

Investigation involves three main elements:

- proof that there is in fact iron deficiency
- detection of possible causes of blood loss
- detection of malabsorption or inadequate iron intake.

In patients with a very low MCV and MCH there is probably no need to measure iron stores directly, though such patients will invariably have a low serum ferritin level. Alternatively, it is possible to measure the serum iron concentration and total iron-binding binding capacity and express these as a percentage of iron saturation; if this is 16% or less it is indicative of iron deficiency.

Detection of blood loss is of major practical importance. No anaemia of any type in old people should be handled without considering blood loss as a possible element in the overall clinical picture.

In the first instance the following issues should be addressed.

- a detailed enquiry into the patient's symptoms, with special reference to the possible sources of bleeding
- a complete physical examination.

Many old people will not readily volunteer facts about their medical history; they will wait to be asked about them directly. Old people are also naturally more reluctant, often simply from modesty, to talk about intimate subjects such as rectal or vaginal bleeding or discharge. It is therefore worth asking direct questions about:

- known previous anaemia
- previous admissions to hospital and any surgical procedures undertaken
- recent changes in bowel habit: constipation, diarrhoea or alternation of these
- rectal or vaginal bleeding or discharge
- haematuria
- special dietary habits and food prejudices
- any drugs that are being taken.

This last question should include 'over-the-counter' purchases such as aspirin, ibuprofen etc. as well as an enquiry into treatment with corticosteroid or prescribed nonsteroidal anti-inflammatory drugs.

Physical examination

Particular points to bear in mind when examining the patient with an iron deficiency anaemia are shown in Figure 12.1. Special attention should be paid to the abdomen; the anus should be inspected and a manual rectal examination performed. If there is a history of vaginal discharge a bimanual and speculum examination of the vagina and cervix should be done.

If there is a history of rectal bleeding or discharge, sigmoidoscopy should be performed after full preparation. A thorough clinical examination of this kind may well give some positive hint of the underlying disease, but it will often be negative.

Investigating the source of blood loss

In elderly people with an iron deficiency anaemia, a decision has to be made as to how far to pursue investigations for the cause of iron loss. To a certain extent this will depend on the patient's overall physical and mental state; in old people who have severe physical or mental disabilities such as a total hemiplegia or advanced dementia, where the

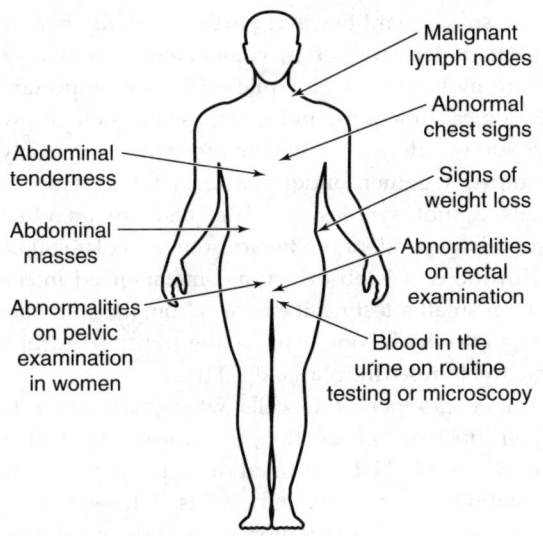

Fig. 12.1 Particular points to remember when looking for the cause of an iron deficiency anaemia.

Image labels:
- Malignant lymph nodes
- Abnormal chest signs
- Signs of weight loss
- Abnormalities on rectal examination
- Blood in the urine on routine testing or microscopy
- Abdominal tenderness
- Abdominal masses
- Abnormalities on pelvic examination in women

Box 12.2 Causes of iron loss in elderly patients

Gastrointestinal blood loss
- Peptic ulcer
- Gastric erosions
- Oesophageal ulceration
- Carcinoma of the stomach, oesophagus or pancreas
- Carcinoma of the colon or rectum
- Angiodysplasia
- Inflammatory bowel disease
- Oesophageal varices
- Haemorrhoids

Genitourinary blood loss
- Primary renal malignancy
- Carcinoma of the bladder
- Carcinoma of the endometrium or cervix
- Chronic haemorrhagic cystitis

---

prognosis is already limited and the quality of life inevitably poor, it is often justifiable to spare the patient the discomfort and distress of endoscopic and radiological examinations of the bowel, though a sensible clinician will need to take the wishes of the patient and the patient's relatives into account.

Testing the stool for occult blood is of limited value. However, if it is persistently negative it is unlikely that the patient has gastrointestinal blood loss. It is very important to test the urine for haematuria.

A small proportion of patients with chronic blood loss have urinary tract disease, particularly malignancy, which may be amenable to treatment. Upper gastrointestinal bleeding is best detected by endoscopy. Bleeding from the colon and terminal ileum can be investigated by colonoscopy or double contrast barium enema, or less invasively by computed tomography (CT) barium examination. The choice of investigation and the order in which several are performed will depend on the patient's symptoms, physical signs and physical state, and the availability of the various methods.

The commonest and most important causes of gastrointestinal and urinary tract blood loss are shown in Box 12.2.

The treatment of iron deficiency anaemia

Treatment of the underlying condition. Of course, this will depend on the nature of the pathology. Some conditions, such as peptic ulceration, can be treated as easily in frail elderly people as in the young. On the other hand, the clinician will need to weigh up the risks and benefits of subjecting an elderly patient to a surgical operation for treatment of, for example, carcinoma of the caecum or hypernephroma.

Iron replacement therapy. The treatment consists, in the great majority of patients, of giving iron-containing drugs by mouth; only rarely is it necessary to resort to intramuscular or intravenous therapy but therapeutic preferences vary and some physicians may prefer the rapidity and certainty of parenteral therapy.

The daily oral dose is between 100 and 150 mg of elemental iron, irrespective of the severity of the anaemia. Failure to obtain the expected response to oral iron occurs in the following circumstances:

- The drug therapy is not being taken properly.
- The amount of iron prescribed is inadequate.
- The underlying pathology has not been treated

or controlled and blood loss continues to outstrip new haemoglobin synthesis.
- Some other disease process has developed during treatment or the original diagnosis was wrong.
- There is malabsorption of the iron.

In patients who have had the cause of their iron loss removed or treated, complete iron replacement should be possible within about 3 months. Some patients in whom iron loss continues will require longer-term maintenance oral iron therapy.

Megaloblastic anaemias

Definition

A megaloblastic anaemia is characterized by the presence in the bone marrow of large nucleated red cell precursors which do not occur in the normal sequence of erythrocyte development. The peripheral blood is macrocytic: that is, the red cells are larger than usual.

It must be remembered that the terms macrocytic and megaloblastic are not synonymous; all megaloblastic anaemias give a macrocytic blood picture, but not all the diseases causing macrocytosis are of megaloblastic origin.

Causes of megaloblastic anaemia in the elderly

For practical purposes megaloblastic anaemia is due to either, vitamin B_{12} or folate deficiency. The B_{12} deficiency is almost always due to pernicious anaemia, a disease caused by the inability of gastric parietal cells to produce a transport protein, the intrinsic factor.

Such patients usually have gastric atrophy and an antiparietal cell auto-antibody can be detected in the blood of the majority. Some patients have had the intrinsic factor-producing part of the stomach removed by extensive gastric surgery. Deficiency of B_{12} is only rarely of strictly nutritional origin. Folate deficiency, on the other hand, most often results from malnutrition, with malabsorption as a common factor.

Sources of folic acid. Folic acid is so named because it occurs in the foliage of plants. As strictly defined chemically, folic acid occurs in nature in only small quantities, but partly or wholly hydrogenated derivates of it, conjugated with one or more molecules of glutamic acid, have important biological functions, and it is these physiologically important derivates which are now commonly lumped together under the term folate. Human cells cannot synthesize folate, and are therefore entirely dependent on dietary sources. Folate taken with the diet is absorbed and metabolized in the upper small intestine; it emerges from the epithelial cells into the bloodstream as the transport form 5 methyl tetrahydrofolic acid (THF).

This can penetrate cells which, according to their biochemical function, transform it into other derivates of THF destined to take part in the metabolism of certain amino acids, in the synthesis of purines, in the initiation of peptide chain synthesis and – a function probably of special importance in the context of megaloblastic anaemia – in the biosynthesis of a deoxyribonucleotide containing thymidine, one of the bases of the nucleic acids.

Sources of vitamin B_{12}. Vitamin B_{12} cannot be synthesized by plants or man, but is widely made by bacteria. After ingestion it is stored in many animal tissues, and human beings depend for supply on their carnivorous diet and on the bacterial contamination of food. The daily requirement is very small, probably only in the region of 2 mcg.

Although vitamin B_{12} deficiency is the commonest cause of megaloblastic anaemia in old age, some cases will be seen which are due to folate deficiency.

The true prevalence of folate deficiency is not certain. In the general population folate deficiency causing severe anaemia is much less common than pernicious anaemia, though in hospital patients in Europe and North America the two are about equally common.

Minor degrees of folate deficiency not clinically expressed as anaemia are probably even commoner, since there is a host of conditions which can cause folate lack. These are summarized in Box 12.3.

The following two points should also be borne in mind in elderly patients with megaloblastic anaemia:

- Some patients will be seen with pernicious anaemia and nutritional folate deficiency.

Box 12.3 Factors associated with folate deficiency

Inadequate intake
- Immobility
- Social isolation
- Apathy
- Poverty
- Undetected depression
- Unusual diets

Malabsorption
- Gluten-sensitive enteropathy
- Dermatitis in herpetiformis
- Small bowel resection
- Chronic pancreatitis

Increased folate utilization
- Neoplasms and reticuloses with rapid primitive cell production

Inhibition of activity
- Drugs such as dihydrofolate reductase inhibitors, methotrexate, trimethoprim

Excessive loss
- Skin diseases with rapid cell turnover, such as psoriasis and exfoliative dermatitis, liver damage and chronic biliary disease

- Iron deficiency may also be present and if not detected and treated will result in an inadequate response to B_{12} and/or folate replacement.

Clinical findings in megaloblastic anaemia

These can be summarized as follows:

- The general features of any severe anaemia will occur, as described above.
- Patients with pernicious anaemia often have glossitis.
- Vitamin B_{12} deficiency occasionally causes subacute combined degeneration of the spinal cord, in which condition the patients will complain of weakness and ataxia of the legs and physical examination will reveal signs of posterior column dysfunction.

- Rare consequences of vitamin B_{12} deficiency include cerebellar dysfunction, peripheral neuropathy and dementia.
- Patients with folate deficiency often have symptoms of the underlying gastrointestinal disease, particularly when there is malabsorption.
- When folate deficiency is severe and of purely nutritional origin, multiple water-soluble vitamin deficiencies will probably coexist, though overt clinical signs of lack of riboflavin, pyridoxine, nicotinic acid or ascorbic acid are very rare in the United Kingdom, Europe, North America and similar societies.

The peripheral blood in megaloblastic anaemia

The typical findings in an uncomplicated case are:

- The mean corpuscular volume (MCV) is increased above 99 fl, and in pernicious anaemia it is often as high as 120–130 fl. In folic acid deficiency it is usually in the range of 100–110 fl. The normal range is 76–99 fl.
- The mean corpuscular Hb concentration (MCHC) is normal.
- The mean corpuscular Hb is increased in proportion with the rise of MCV. The normal range is 27–32 picograms.
- The peripheral blood film shows large red cells of normal or dense colour and these are often polychromatic. (Blue colour is due to persistence of cytoplasmic RNA.) The cells are more variable than normal in both size and shape; pear-shaped red cells are common.
- The white blood cell count (normal range 4 000–11 000 per mm²) is usually reduced. There is an absolute fall in polymorphs, but those present are often hypersegmented.
- The platelet count is either normal or reduced; if it is very low, the prognosis is less good.
- Serum ferritin is normal or high unless there is concurrent iron deficiency.

If all these features are present in the peripheral blood, a provisional diagnosis of megaloblastic anaemia can be made, but proof requires an examination of the bone marrow, which will show hypercellularity, the characteristic megaloblasts and profuse reticulo-endothelial iron.

Further investigations

There are two aspects to these, as follows:

- The cause of the megaloblastic anaemia can be verified by measuring serum vitamin B_{12} and the folate concentration of serum and red cells. This will enable a clinician to differentiate pure deficiency states of B_{12} or folate, or a mixed deficiency.
- If it is thought that a general malabsorption syndrome is contributing, the patient will need to be investigated accordingly for its cause.

The treatment of megaloblastic anaemia

Pernicious anaemia.   The treatment consists of intramuscular injections of vitamin B_{12}, given for the rest of the patient's life, and this fact must be explained clearly to both the patient and relatives.

The preferred drug is hydroxocobalamin, which is given as 1000 mcg i.m. on alternate days for 1 week then 250 mcg weekly until the blood count is normal. The maintenance dosage is 1000 mcg every 3 months.

The patient should be kept under review for the first 3 months of therapy. Failure to sustain the response to therapy can be due to one of the following factors:

- Injections are not being given, or not in adequate amounts.
- Iron deficiency coexists; the serum ferritin concentration will then be low, and the patient will require treatment with oral iron and investigation for the cause of the iron deficiency.
- The diagnosis is wrong and the patient has some other reason for macrocytosis, such as hypothyroidism.
- There is coexisting folate deficiency, though this will usually have been detected at the initial investigation.

Folate should not be given alone before giving vitamin B_{12} therapy to patients with pernicious anaemia as there is a risk of precipitating subacute combined degeneration of the spinal cord.

Treatment of folic acid deficiency anaemia. This can be summarized as follows:

- Folic acid replacement therapy by mouth in an initial dose of 5 mg t.d.s.
- Treating malabsorption if present, including replacement therapy for any other nutrients in which the patient is deficient.
- When oral therapy is not practical, folic acid can be given by i.m. injection, 15 mg o.d. If it is a purely nutritional deficiency of folate then other vitamins are also likely to be lacking and should be replaced by a multivitamin preparation. Replacement of body folate stores normally occurs within a few days, but if the factors causing folate deficiency are likely to recur, prophylactic treatment is continued. Iron deficiency can coexist with folate deficiency just as in pernicious anaemia.

The anaemia of chronic disease

A wide range of chronic inflammatory conditions and neoplasms can cause a nonspecific moderate anaemia through mechanisms which are only partially understood.

Some examples of such conditions are contained in Box 12.4. However, in old people the three most important mechanisms are chronic infection, chronic renal failure and rheumatoid arthritis. We will look at these in a little more detail.

Box 12.4 Some important chronic conditions causing 'anaemia of chronic disease'

- Chronic infection (see text)
- Chronic renal failure (see text)
- Chronic inflammatory joint disease (see text)
- Any long-term inflammation
- Connective tissue disorders
- Malignancy

Chronic infection

Anaemia is often associated with common chronic infections in old age. Examples would include chronic pyelonephritis, infected leg ulcers, indolent soft tissue infections, infected pressure sores, diverticulitis, tuberculosis and many others less common. Only severe infections and those of long standing will cause anaemia, and even then the blood disorder is usually mild to moderate. The underlying mechanisms are complex and poorly understood, but the three main factors include disturbed iron metabolism, impaired haemoglobin synthesis and depression of bone marrow function. The red cells are normocytic and normochromic in most cases and patients who are found to be microcytic, macrocytic or hypochromatic might need to be investigated further for other causes of anaemia.

The anaemia of chronic infection does not respond to oral iron therapy and is best treated by detecting and eradicating the underlying infection if possible.

Patients may need temporary support by a blood transfusion, and if an untreatable infection is present this may need to be repeated. The Hb level at which transfusion should be given will depend very much on the clinical context, though patients usually benefit symptomatically from transfusion if their haemoglobin concentration has fallen below 90 gm/1.

Chronic renal failure

Patients with chronic renal failure are invariably anaemic. The most important mechanism is failure of the renal production of erythropoietin which is essential for maintaining normal haemoglobin levels.

Toxin-induced bone marrow suppression is probably also an important mechanism in these circumstances. The anaemia is normochromic and normocytic, and it is rarely severe unless the glomerular filtration rate falls below 15 ml/min., after which the depression of haemoglobin correlates well with the reduction in glomerular filtration rate. Treatment may not be necessary if there is only a moderate stable anaemia. More severe anaemia can be treated with injections of erythropoietin, and it is important not to overlook the pos-

sibility of a coexisting specific cause for the anaemia.

Rheumatoid arthritis

Rheumatoid arthritis is common in elderly people and is often accompanied by anaemia. Two types of blood disturbance are recognized:

- Most patients will have a normocytic anaemia which is either normochromic or slightly hypochromic.
- Folate utilization is high in active rheumatoid disease so some patients present with a megaloblastic anaemia.
- The normochromic anaemia is usually seen in patients with active rheumatoid arthritis and is associated with indices of disease activity such as a high erythrocyte sedimentation rate or high C-reactive protein level. It is worth remembering that a great many of these patients are also taking drugs which can cause anaemia such as nonsteroidal antiinflammatory drugs and corticosteroids, which can cause gastrointestinal bleeding; immunosuppressive drugs which sometimes depress bone marrow; and drugs which interfere with folate metabolism, such as methotrexate.

The anaemia in rheumatoid arthritis does not usually respond to iron therapy unless there is a coexisting iron deficiency state.

Corticosteroid therapy for the rheumatoid disease is usually associated with an improvement in haemoglobin concentration. Patients receiving methotrexate should take a folic acid supplement.

A small number of patients who become very anaemic may require blood transfusion, particularly to tide them over a period of intense rheumatoid disease activity.

The myelodysplastic syndrome

Another important cause of anaemia seen exclusively in elderly patients is caused by myelodysplasia. This is a condition of bone marrow stem cells and there are a number of subgroups under the general heading of myelodysplasia. Reduction in all blood cell lines may be seen; the condition is premalignant and may transform to myeloid leukaemia, though patients with the condition also succumb to infection if they are neutropenic or haemorrhage if their platelet count is low. The anaemia seen may be normochromic or macrocytic and does not respond to treatment with haematinic agents unless there is coexisting haematinic deficiency.

Patients with the more benign forms of the disease can often be maintained for several years by occasional blood transfusions to top up the haemoglobin level. It is important not to make the diagnosis without thorough investigation, which must include expert examination of the bone marrow.

Heart disease

Introduction

In Europe and North America heart disease accounts for about one-third of deaths, and for a large amount of morbidity and disability in old age. The most important and common cause is myocardial ischaemia, closely followed by hypertensive heart disease, and then by mixed cases where both these diseases are present. Furthermore, the advent of modern drug therapy for cardiac failure has resulted in a large number of old people being supported for a long time, often years, before they succumb to the terminal phase of severe heart failure. Many of these patients require close monitoring and are frail and dependent, which results in a considerable strain on financial and human resources.

The subject of cardiac disease in old age is a very large one and is dealt with in a number of specialized textbooks.

In this chapter we will concentrate on the common cardiac conditions in old age, and emphasize some of those aspects of cardiac disease in the frail elderly which are not always covered in the standard textbooks.

Changes in cardiac physiology with age

The very old myocardium often shows brown atrophy. The pigmentation is caused by the accumulation of lipofuscin in myocardial cells, though this is probably of no physiological importance. At autopsy, in the absence of preceding pathological conditions causing myocardial hypertrophy, there is a tendency for the heart weight to fall in old age, and this seems to be part and parcel of the overall fall in lean body mass as age advances. Fibrotic patches within the myocardium are common in old age; some of these may be due to previous myocardial infarction and the presence of such changes correlates well with the severity of coronary artery atherosclerosis. Amyloid change is also common in old age and has been found in up to 12% of patients over the age of 80 at autopsy.

When the left ventricle is extensively involved, cardiac performance is compromised and heart failure eventually occurs, although this is not common. Like fibrosis secondary to ischaemic heart disease, cardiac amyloidosis probably ought not to be regarded as a true age-related process, and its cause is unknown. Age-related changes also occur in the cardiac conducting system and the number of cells in the sino-atrial node decreases.

The control of heart rate

The mean resting heart rate changes little with age. However, the intrinsic rate of the sino-atrial node falls in old age. Some individuals have a considerably higher resting pulse rate when they are older. Such people have often previously had very low resting heart rates as a result of physical training, and this vagally mediated reduction in heart rate wanes in old age. The maximum heart rate achievable during exercise falls during old age, so that few individuals over the age of 80 can generate a sinus tachycardia of more than 140 p.m. Of course, a reduced heart rate response is one of the factors limiting cardiac output in old age.

Cardiac output

Most studies of the resting cardiac output have shown a decline in old age, and the achievable rise in cardiac output during exercise is certainly less in the old adult compared with the young, even in the absence of overt cardiac disease.

Though oxygen consumption falls in old age, the even greater fall in cardiac output leads to a higher arteriovenous oxygen difference than in the young, especially during exercise. At rest, the fall in cardiac output is mainly due to a lower stroke volume. The mean systolic blood pressure rises with age while resting cardiac output falls.

This, of course, is due to the rise in peripheral vascular resistance. The gradual rise in systolic and diastolic blood pressure seen in cross-sectional studies in Western industrial countries might not be a true ageing change but the consequence of a complex interaction between diet, body weight, salt intake and a relatively sedentary lifestyle.

It is noteworthy that very little increase in either systolic or diastolic blood pressure between young adult life and old age is observed in peoples whose lifestyle is physically active, whose salt consumption is low and whose body weight remains stable throughout adult life; examples include the pygmies of central Africa, the bushmen of the Kalahari and the indigenous peoples of the forests of Brazil.

The Starling curve in old age

The decline in cardiac reserve is probably best illustrated by the Starling curve relating cardiac output to left ventricular end-diastolic pressure. Thus in the hypothetical case shown in Figure 13.1 it can be seen that the maximum achievable cardiac output before cardiac failure occurs falls between the ages of 25 and 60, and even more so from 60 to 90. Therefore, an event such as a myocardial infarction, which displaces the curve downwards, is more likely to result in cardiac decompensation in the very old heart.

This is a very good example of how reserves of function fall with age, and where relatively small superimposed pathological insults can result in physiological failure. Therefore, physicians must remember that relatively small amounts of damage

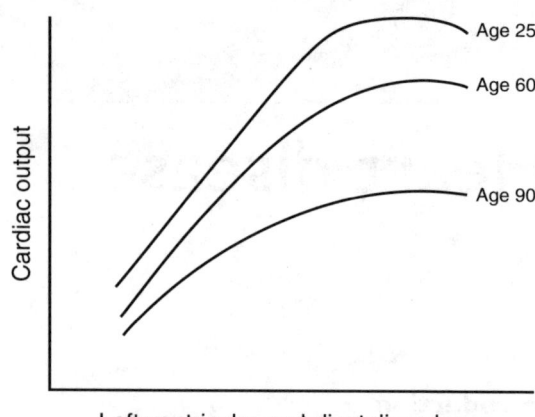

Fig. 13.1 The Starling curve in people of different ages.

to the aged myocardium can result in severe heart failure, and that conversely, steps taken to salvage small amounts of myocardium during acute myocardial infarction can be extremely beneficial in old age. By the same token, the aged myocardium is less able to tolerate episodes of sustained tachycardia, thyrotoxicosis, severe systemic hypertension, pulmonary embolism etc. when compared with a younger heart.

Ageing and cardiovascular fitness

One of the most useful measures of overall cardiovascular fitness is the maximum oxygen consumption ($\dot{V}O_2$ max) during exercise testing. As shown in Figure 13.2, cross-sectional studies of healthy adult

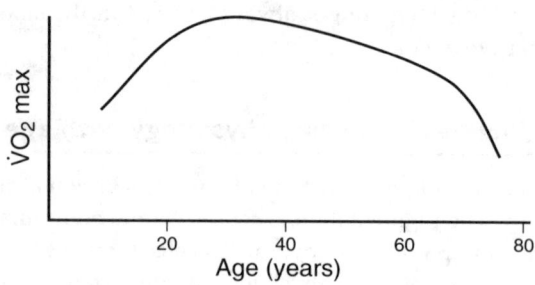

Fig. 13.2 Cross-sectional studies of healthy people in industrialized societies show a decline in the maximum achievable oxygen consumption ($\dot{V}O_2$ max) from the age of 25, with a steep decline after 65.

Europeans has shown an approximately linear fall in the mean maximum oxygen consumption from the age of around 25–65.

However, when individuals from the same society who take regular exercise are studied it is found that between the ages of 25 and 60 the decline in maximum oxygen uptake is much less than the average. This is shown in figure 13.3. It is well known that fitness training at any age results in a rise in maximum oxygen consumption and the resulting improvement in this aspect of cardio respiratory reserve is a strong point in favour of taking regular exercise throughout life; this may be one of the reasons why older individuals who exercise regularly are more likely to survive a myocardial infarction.

Clinical features of heart disease in old age

The important major symptoms of chest pain, breathlessness, orthopnoea, paroxysmal nocturnal dyspnoea and exercise intolerance are much the same in old people as they are in the young. Therefore, we will not dwell on them in this chapter. More importantly, it must be remembered that aged people who suffer cardiac events which cause a fall in cardiac output, such as a myocardial infarction, atrial fibrillation or worsening of cardiac failure, will often present with major geriatric problems which eclipse the usual cardiac symptoms.

For example, if a patient develops atrial fibrillation the resulting drop in cardiac output may pre-

sent as confusion, falls or even incontinence and the patient will then not be likely to complain spontaneously of reduced exercise tolerance or breathlessness on exertion. It is sometimes said that old people are less likely to experience typical cardiac chest pain with myocardial infarction and angina.

There is some evidence that silent myocardial ischaemia is commoner in old people, though this must not be regarded as the rule, and the majority of people over the age of 75 with significant myocardial ischaemia or myocardial infarction will complain of cardiac chest pain. However, it must be remembered that other symptoms may also be present; this can confuse the issue, and patients who become acutely confused are sometimes unable to report their chest pain, while those with dementia may not remember it.

Some physical signs become less reliable with age, and a good example is the presence of basal lung crackles. In old people basal lung crackles cannot be relied upon as a sign of pulmonary oedema since they are so prevalent amongst old people irrespective of their cardiovascular status.

Systolic murmurs also deserve a mention in this context. A systolic murmur is a common finding in an old person and it is often quite difficult, on clinical grounds, to decide whether significant valve pathology is present or not. In the first instance it is necessary to try to determine whether the murmur is arising from the aortic valve or from reflux through the mitral valve, and the main distinguishing features are outlined in Box 13.1.

> ### Box 13.1 Important clinical features of aortic and mitral systolic murmurs
>
> **Aortic systolic murmur**
> — Has typical ejection or 'diamond-shaped' sound, maximal in mid-systole
> — Heard well in aortic area
> — Radiates to the carotid area
>
> **Mitral systolic murmur**
> — Often pansystolic
> — Sometimes late-systolic
> — Heard well at the apex
> — Radiates to the left axilla

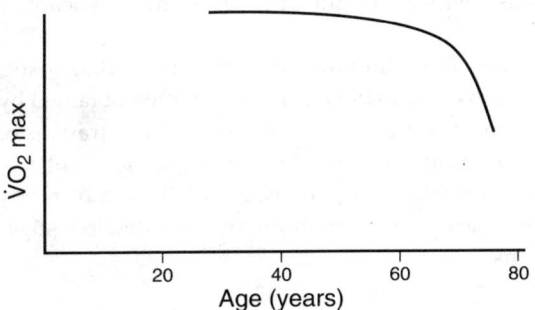

Fig. 13.3 Individuals who exercise regularly can maintain their V̇O₂ max until the inevitable decline after the age of 60.

It is now known that assessment of the severity of aortic stenosis and mitral valve reflux by auscultation is very unreliable. Therefore, if such murmurs are discovered, and particularly if a patient has symptoms which might be caused by valvular heart disease, the severity of the stenosis, or reflux, needs to be assessed by echocardiography. Aortic stenosis is very common in old people in Europe and North America and is most commonly due to degenerative changes with calcification of the aortic wall and valve cusps, though in some developing countries postrheumatic valvular stenosis is still relatively common.

Modern surgical techniques now enable old people with severe aortic stenosis to benefit from valve replacement surgery, and age itself should not be a bar to referral for surgical intervention. Mitral incompetence in the elderly is usually caused by dilatation of the left ventricle with distortion of the mitral valve ring in patients with heart failure; rheumatic mitral valve disease is now relatively uncommon in the developed parts of the world, though it is still occasionally seen. Other causes of mitral incompetence include calcification of the mitral annulus, rupture of the chordae tendinae, prolapse of a degenerative posterior mitral cusp into the left atrium during systole, and, very rarely, left atrial myxoma.

Symptoms and presentation of myocardial infarction in old age

Myocardial infarction is a common and often catastrophic event in old people. However, recent research has shown that active treatment of myocardial infarction with modern therapy, including thrombolysis, has an even better influence on prognosis in old people than in those of middle age.

The reason for this is not entirely clear but may be due in part to better collateral blood supply to the myocardium in old people and partly due to the fact, as mentioned above, that salvaging small amounts of myocardium in old age can make the difference between having an adequate cardiac output or lapsing into cardiac decompensation.

Therefore, it is very important to make the diagnosis quickly and to take immediate action.

About 60% of elderly people with myocardial infarction give a history of some chest pain, and about 90% will have either chest pain, dyspnoea, syncope or a combination of these. Other modes of presentation in old age include:

- the development of acute brain failure
- persistent severe hypotension
- arterial embolism from a thrombosis formed over the infarcted endocardium; the embolus may pass to the brain causing a stroke or to noncerebral arteries causing a variety of clinical syndromes
- vomiting and weakness
- other geriatric problems such as falls and incontinence.

Finally, some myocardial infarctions in the aged are completely silent and are discovered only by electrocardiography. It is likely that such silent myocardial infarctions are equally prevalent in patients of middle age. However, some apparently silent myocardial infarctions in old age are due to symptoms having been forgotten in patients with dementia.

Investigations

The electrocardiogram (ECG) is not intrinsically altered by age, and the electrocardiographic features of myocardial infarction are the same in older people as they are in the middle-aged. An electrocardiogram should be performed immediately when an old person presents with an illness which might be due to myocardial infarction.

The ECG findings are sometimes diagnostic, though confirmatory evidence is often obtained by demonstrating a rise in the blood concentrations of myocardial enzymes released as a result of myocardial damage or necrosis. It is only rarely necessary to perform more sophisticated investigations.

Management of myocardial infarction in old age

The student is referred to standard textbooks of cardiology and acute medicine for details of the management of myocardial infarction. However, it is very important to emphasize in this chapter that the evidence from extensive trials has demonstrated that age alone should not be a bar to active treatment of myocardial infarction in old age, and that the full range of therapies, including thrombolysis and coronary care unit support and monitoring, should be made available to people of all ages unless there are coexisting pathological conditions which would discourage the physician from treating the patient vigorously.

Angina

The diagnosis and treatment of angina pectoris is the same in old people as in the middle-aged and young. However, the diagnosis is sometimes more difficult to make in an old person, particularly in patients with cognitive impairment and those where there is a wide range of symptoms from multiple coexisting pathologies.

Furthermore, some old people have their exercise tolerance limited by a number of factors simultaneously and ischaemic cardiac chest pain may be just one of these. For example, a patient with ischaemic heart disease, chronic airflow limitation and rheumatoid arthritis may be limited by chest pain and breathlessness on some occasions and by pain in the knees and feet on others. The clinician needs to be very wary of these confounding factors when assessing angina in such patients.

Cardiac failure

Like myocardial infarction, acute cardiac failure is managed in old people by the same methods used in younger people. However, there are some differences in the approach required for the management of chronic cardiac failure. Although the majority of old people with chronic heart failure will have underlying ischaemic heart disease, it is important to identify and treat potentially reversible causes of cardiac failure, some of which are shown in Box 13.2.

Box 13.2 Potentially treatable causes of chronic cardiac failure in old age

- Hypertension
- Valvular disease when this is amenable to surgical correction
- Drug side-effects, particularly high-dose betablocker treatment
- Cardiac arrhythmias
- Multiple pulmonary embolism
- Anaemia
- Thyrotoxicosis
- Pericardial effusion

Furthermore it must be emphasized that the elderly patient with chronic heart failure might present with the typical symptoms of effort dysponea, orthopnoea and paroxysmal nocturnal dyspnoea, but is also very likely to present with nonspecific symptoms such as weakness, tiredness, inability to cope and fatigue.

Furthermore, some elderly patients with chronic heart failure do not present to their physicians until some other event, such as an episode of pneumonia, makes matters worse and results in further decompensation.

Treatment of chronic heart failure

Moderate doses of a loop diuretic should be given to all patients, and the dose can be adjusted according to the clinical response. There is a body of evidence to suggest that further symptomatic improvement can be gained by adding an angiotensin converting enzyme (ACE) inhibitor, though it is not clear whether these agents improve the prognosis in cardiac failure in the same way as they do after myocardial infarction.

Care must be taken when prescribing ACE inhibitors because of the tendency for patients to develop hypotension, hyponatraemia and a rise in blood urea. Most patients taking a moderate dose of a loop diuretic do not require potassium supplements providing their diet is reasonable, though some do become hypokalaemic and will require a potassium supplement once other causes of hypokalaemia have been excluded.

Diuretic combinations which include potassium-sparing agents have a tendency to cause severe hyponatraemia in old people and should be avoided. Other aspects of the treatment of chronic heart failure in old people are the same as in younger people and will not be dealt with in detail in this chapter.

Orthostatic hypotension

A large fall of blood pressure on standing is a common cause of symptoms in old people, can lead to substantial disability, and is often amenable to treatment if properly assessed and managed. Patients with postural hypotension usually present with one or more of the following clinical problems:

- a feeling of faintness on standing
- falls, often accompanied by an aura of faintness
- syncope
- a feeling of weakness in all four limbs on standing.

These symptoms will appear on standing and will disappear when the patient is lying down. There is a tendency for the symptoms to be worse in a hot environment, or after a bath or large meal. Occasionally, elderly men complain of similar symptoms during or after micturition, and this is usually due to straining to pass urine in a patient with prostatic hypertrophy with a consequent reduction in venous return during the phase of high intrathoracic and intra-abdominal pressure.

Confirmation of postural hypotension

If the condition is suspected, confirmation of the diagnosis is a relatively simple matter. In gross cases the radial pulse will become imperceptible on standing, though the usual means of confirming the diagnosis is by taking the blood pressure in the lying position and then to repeat this immediately on standing and about 2 minutes after standing.

The normal response to assuming the erect posture is first a brief dip of both the systolic and the diastolic pressures; the stabilized response is a slight rise of diastolic pressure with little change in the systolic pressure, and the resultant drop in pulse pressure is accompanied by a slight rise in pulse rate. The patient is asked to lie supine for at least 5 minutes before the first blood pressure measurement is taken.

The majority of old people show the same blood pressure response to standing as the young. Arbitrarily, a fall in the systolic blood pressure of 20 mmHg is taken as being significant, but more important than the actual figure is whether there are associated symptoms.

The causes of postural hypotension

These are shown in Box 13.3.

Box 13.3 Causes of postural hypotension in old age

- Drugs, particularly antihypertensive drugs, diuretics, phenothiazine tranquillizers and tricyclic antidepressants
- Hypovolaemia, due to dehydration, bleeding, sodium depletion or adrenal insufficiency
- Severe bacterial and viral infection
- Low cardiac output states
- Pooling of blood in the lower limbs due to severe varicose veins
- Prolonged bed rest
- Autonomic dysfunction, idiopathic or secondary to various diseases which can damage neurological tissue, of which diabetes mellitus is the most common

Note Many old people have a combination of these factors.

Drugs are probably the most common cause of postural hypotension in old people and it is essential to find out what medication an affected patient is currently taking. The sensible course is to withdraw all but the essential drugs and observe the effect on blood pressure, though it is often possible by looking at the timing of prescriptions and the timing of the onset of symptoms to isolate and identify the offending drug, particularly when this is one of the drugs which is commonly associated with postural hypotension.

Investigation

The details of investigations will depend on the clinical picture and on what the underlying mechanism is thought to be. In patients who are thought to have autonomic dysfunction it is helpful to perform tests of cardiovascular reflexes. Recent research has shown that the blood pressure response to 70° head-up tilting is the most reliable way of testing these responses, though various other methods have also been validated.

Patients who complain of syncope should also be tested for carotid sinus hypersensitivity by performing carotid sinus massage while blood pressure and pulse rate are monitored continuously. This will detect bradycardic and hypotensive responses with a good degree of reliability.

Treatment

Treatment is usually only successful when some cause can be identified and removed. This is relatively straightforward in patients with drug-induced hypotension, dehydration, hypovolaemia or adrenal failure. In such cases it is a relatively simple matter of adjusting therapy and treating the underlying causes. Other forms of postural hypotension are more difficult to treat, though some of the following approaches to treatment are helpful:

- Patients with severe varicose veins are often helped by full-length compression stockings.
- Patients with mild to moderate idiopathic autonomic neuropathy are usually best treated by a combination of lower limb compression stockings, low-dose fludrocortisone therapy and a high caffeine intake. Care has to be taken with fludrocortisone as it can cause severe salt and water retention and worsen heart failure.
- Some patients have been successfully treated by a combination of tyramine and a monoamine oxidase inhibitor, though monitoring therapy is extremely difficult and the patients tend to have episodes of severe hypertension.

- Postural hypotension occurring after a severe acute illness, such as pneumonia, influenza or prolonged bed rest, is often helped by gradual postural retraining, during which the patient is placed in progressively more erect positions over a number of days until the cardiovascular reflexes improve sufficiently to maintain blood pressure in the upright position.

When treating patients with idiopathic postural hypotension it is sensible to aim for sufficient improvement to help symptoms rather than to give excessive therapy in a vain attempt to normalize the standing blood pressure.

Those patients with very severe postural hypotension which does not respond to the measures outlined will often need to adapt to a wheelchair existence and be helped to make the necessary adjustments to their lifestyle, living environment and domestic arrangements.

Hypertension in the elderly

When large groups of patients are studied in the industrialized countries of Europe and North America, both the systolic and diastolic blood pressures continue to rise throughout adult life until about the age of 65, after which there is no overall further increase. About 5% of men and women over 65 will have a systolic blood pressure exceeding 200 mmHg and a diastolic of 100 mmHg or more, in the absence of treatment. Many patients with blood pressure levels as high as this feel well and have no symptoms, though we now know that, without intervention, such high levels of blood pressure predispose these patients like their younger counterparts to a number of common complications including stroke, myocardial infarction and hypertensive heart failure.

It is not always possible to rely on isolated blood pressure measurement, though it must be borne in mind that all the trials of the efficacy of intervention have been based on ordinary sphygmomanometer readings; in some individuals it is necessary to obtain further evidence of genuine hypertension before giving drug treatment, particularly when there is reason to believe that the patient becomes tense and anxious during a consultation.

Therefore, the following factors can be helpful when trying to decide whether blood pressure measurements are indicative of sustained hypertension in an individual:

- evidence of left ventricular hypertrophy on the electrocardiogram
- evidence of concentric left ventricular hypertrophy on echocardiography
- evidence of target organ damage, such as deteriorating renal function and hypertensive retinopathy
- evidence on 24-hour blood pressure (BP) monitoring of sustained very high blood pressures, or loss of the normal physiological fall in blood pressure during sleep.

Patients with very high blood pressures, such as a sustained diastolic pressure of 130 mmHg or more, should be considered to be medical emergencies, as would be the case for the younger patient. Patients with this level of sustained hypertension are at particular risk of developing heart failure, renal failure and cerebral haemorrhage, and careful, controlled reduction in blood pressure is essential.

At what level should hypertension be treated in people over the age of 65?

There is now a substantial amount of evidence to show that a reduction in both fatal and nonfatal myocardial infarction, and in stroke can be achieved by treating older people with systolic blood pressures persistently above 160 mmHg and/or diastolic pressures consistently above 90 mmHg.

The case for the benefits of such treatment is now well established for people in the so-called young elderly group, that is 65–80 years, though there is also some evidence that benefit also occurs in people over the age of 80.

Treatment

Because of the risks of side-effects, particularly postural hypotension, elderly people require a particularly cautious approach to antihypertensive therapy and the blood pressure reduction target should be modest and achieved gradually.

Most patients with mild to moderate hypertension can obtain a reasonable reduction in blood pressure with 2.5 mg of bendrofluazide per day, and the trial evidence supports this. Some patients may need additional therapy, and the choice of drug will to a large extent be determined by the need to treat any coexisting conditions. Therefore, for example, a patient with hypertension and heart failure could sensibly be treated with an ACE inhibitor, whereas a patient with hypertension and angina might be better receiving a betablocker such as atenolol or calcium channel antagonist such as amlodipine.

Clinicians should not be afraid to use betablockers in elderly people when there are no absolute contraindications, since there is no firm evidence that betablocker side-effects, particularly with low to moderate doses, are any more prevalent in elderly people than in their younger counterparts. Occasionally, other antihypertensive agents will be required, depending on the clinical context.

The special liability of old people to digitalis intoxication

Digitalis intoxication is common in old people and is probably underdiagnosed. The reason for this is the widespread use of digoxin in the treatment of atrial fibrillation and cardiac failure. However, other factors are concerned in the prevalence of intoxication from this drug. Firstly, digoxin is often prescribed in aged patients in a dose more appropriate to younger people. In old people the lean body mass, in which the digoxin is distributed, is reduced, and myocardial concentrations of digoxin tend therefore to be high. Secondly, digoxin is excreted only by the kidneys, whose function is often reduced in old age with a corresponding risk of drug accumulation.

Therefore, effective digitalization in a 25-year-old man weighing 100 kg with normal renal function might require a dose as high as 0.25 mg twice daily for maintenance therapy, whereas a dose as small as 0.125 mg daily may cause serious digoxin toxicity in an 80-year-old woman weighing 40 kg with poor renal function.

In the first instance the detection of digoxin toxicity depends on clinical observation. The patients may present very nonspecifically but the following symptoms and signs are very helpful:

- Patients often complain of nausea, poor appetite, a feeling of ill health and generalized weakness.
- The pulse rate is usually below 60 and pulsus bigeminus may be present. However, a very wide range of arrhythmias can occur in the context of digoxin toxicity, including tachyarrhythmias.
- The patient is likely to show a very marked digitalis effect on the ST segments on the electrocardiogram.
- Digoxin toxicity should be particularly suspected in patients who are known to have poor renal function and in those who are found to be hypokalaemic and who are therefore rendered more sensitive to the effects of digoxin.

Digoxin assay techniques are now widely available in many countries and the clinician should be ready to measure the digoxin concentration in any patient in whom digoxin toxicity is a possibility.

Despite its toxic side-effects, digoxin remains a useful drug in patients of all ages for controlling the ventricular response in atrial fibrillation and there has been a recent renaissance in its use in cardiac failure in patients with sinus rhythm, based on evidence from trials in Europe. When prescribing digoxin it is better in the first instance to err on the side of low rather than high dosage, to use nomograms which take into account age, serum creatinine and body weight when determining the loading dose and maintenance dose, and to use serum digoxin measurements to ensure that the patient is not drifting into the toxic range.

Disturbances of heart rate and rhythm in old age

As ischaemic heart disease is so prevalent in old people, disturbances of heart rate and rhythm are common problems of practical management.

In general, their clinical significance is much the same as in younger adults, though there are a number of special aspects in old age which need to be borne in mind:

- Cerebral blood flow is often reduced in older people with cerebrovascular disease, and adapts less rapidly and less completely to changes in cardiac output. Therefore very fast and very slow heart rates, accompanied by a fall in blood pressure, are important causes of blackouts, episodes of faintness and acute confusion in elderly people.
- Reduced myocardial reserve is often present as a result of ageing and ischaemic heart disease. Consequently, old people with sustained tachyarrhythmias lapse very readily into cardiac failure.

Atrial fibrillation

This is by far the commonest significant arrhythmia in old age. Although sometimes perceived as a benign arrhythmia, atrial fibrillation should be taken seriously in old age for the following reasons:

- In atrial fibrillation, patients lose the augmentation of cardiac output gained by atrial systole. The reduction in cardiac output can be critical in old people and lead to symptoms such as fatigue, exercise intolerance, confusion and breathlessness.
- Patients with chronic atrial fibrillation sometimes develop thrombi in the left atrium which can embolize to the cerebral circulation and other parts of the body.
- If the ventricular response to atrial fibrillation is very fast, cardiac output can be compromised, and the patient may develop overt cardiac failure, or complain of other symptoms such as angina.
- Various aspects of atrial fibrillation can be treated with definite benefit in old age.

Causes of atrial fibrillation

In atrial fibrillation the atrial myocardium is not paced from the sino-atrial node or any other single focus; chaotic discharge takes place and effective atrial contraction is lost. In the majority of people the main predisposing factor is ischaemic heart disease.

Acute atrial fibrillation may be a presenting feature of a number of acute medical illnesses including infection, pulmonary embolism, myocardial infarction, thyrotoxicosis and electrolyte disturbances, and a result of the toxic effects of drugs, particularly digoxin and drugs with sympathomimetic activity.

Treatment of atrial fibrillation

The approach to treatment falls into three main categories; these are treatment of any predisposing causes when possible, treatment of the rhythm disturbance itself, and prophylaxis against the formation of atrial thrombi.

Treatment of the underlying cause. The important issue here is to be certain that no treatable underlying causes are missed. Patients with acute atrial fibrillation in the context of, for example, pneumonia clearly need to have treatment for the pneumonia at the same time as the arrhythmia is being dealt with.

Those with thyrotoxicosis will need appropriate management of the endocrine abnormality and it is very important not to miss some of the subtler underlying causes such as pulmonary embolism.

The details of the treatment of these conditions is dealt with in major textbooks.

Treatment of the arrhythmia. Patients with acute atrial fibrillation sometimes spontaneously revert to sinus rhythm when the underlying cause is treated. Meanwhile, if the ventricular response is fast, particularly when it is greater than 100 p.m., the rate should be controlled with appropriate medication.

Digoxin is suitable if used carefully and other appropriate drugs are amiodarone and sotalol. In those subjects with acute atrial fibrillation which does not return to sinus rhythm with removal of the underlying cause and drug therapy, there is good evidence that even in old age a large proportion of such patients can be successfully brought back into sinus rhythm by direct current (DC) cardioversion. The usual precaution is to anticoagulate the patient for about 4 weeks to avoid thromboembolism at the time of cardioversion.

Prophylaxis against thromboembolism. Patients who show a left atrial diameter of greater than 5 cm (2 inches) on echocardiography can rarely be converted permanently to sinus rhythm. Patients with known chronic atrial fibrillation are less likely to be successfully cardioverted. Such patients require adequate control of the ventricular rate with drugs and anticoagulation to reduce the risks of thromboembolic stroke. There is good evidence to show that the risk of stroke is reduced by 60% by moderate anticoagulation with warfarin in patients with atrial fibrillation. A lesser reduction in risk is obtained with aspirin (about 30%), though in patients over the age of 80, warfarin and aspirin appear to confer about the same amount of protection.

Physiological sinus bradycardia

Some healthy old people have a persistent regular heart rate as slow as 50 b.p.m. When this is known to be longstanding and there are no symptoms and a normal ECG, there is no need for any further investigation or action.

Other important bradyarrhythmias in old age

Some important causes of bradyarrhythmias in old people are contained in Box 13.4.

> ### Box 13.4 Common causes of bradycardia in old people
>
> - Drugs, particularly betablockers, digoxin and diltiazem
> - Sino-atrial block
> - Second-degree heart block
> - Complete heart block
> - Sick sinus syndrome
> - Physiological sinus bradycardia
> - Hypothyroidism
> - Raised intracranial pressure
> - Liver failure

Drug-induced bradycardia is most often caused by betablocking drugs, and this cause is obvious when the patient is taking oral betablockers for angina or hypertension. However, it is important to remember that betablocker eye drops can also cause bradycardia, particularly if the patient is taking an excessive amount because of a poor dropper technique, or when the individual is highly sensitive to betablockers. Digoxin toxicity is also a common cause of bradycardia, and as the drug is most frequently used to slow the ventricular response in atrial fibrillation, the cardiac rhythm is often an irregular bradycardia, though this may become regular if the patient develops complete heart block. Patients with disease of the sino-atrial node will have an intermittent bradycardia, with P waves usually present on the ECG, and those with second-degree heart block will have characteristic ECG changes.

In complete heart block, transmission of supraventricular (SV) impulses through the atrioventricular (AV) node is absent; the ventricles are then driven by a new focus arising spontaneously in the ventricular myocardium. The resulting idioventricular rate is very slow, often in the 35–45 b.p.m. range.

The condition can often be recognized clinically by the very slow heart rate, the presence of cannon waves in the jugular veins (caused by the atria contracting against fortuitously closed AV valves) and audible atrial contractions in the long intervals between ventricular contractions.

The ECG reveals regular P waves occurring at a higher rate than and independently of the QRS complexes. The QRS complex, usually prolonged in duration and deformed in shape, resembles a ventricular ectopic beat, because it usually arises far below the division of the bundle of His. These characteristic ECG changes are illustrated in Figure 13.4. Complete heart block is a serious matter; it will often cause Stokes-Adams attacks and hence

blackouts and falls with the attendant risk of physical injury and occasionally sudden death.

The treatment of complete heart block, sino-atrial disease with bradycardia, second-degree heart block with severe bradycardia and atrial fibrillation with severe bradycardia is with the insertion of a permanent cardiac pacemaker.

Unless there is serious coexisting pathology, such as terminal malignancy, old people of any age can benefit enormously from a pacemaker which should be inserted without delay once treatable underlying causes have been excluded.

The sick sinus syndrome

Patients with this condition usually present with episodes of sinus bradycardia and supraventricular tachycardias which may be interspersed with long periods of normal sinus rhythm. The condition tends to become gradually worse and the patients most commonly complain of faintness or blackouts during the bradycardic episodes.

The condition can sometimes be detected on ordinary electrocardiography, though 24-hour ECG monitoring is more likely to establish the diagnosis. This is a serious condition which can cause considerable morbidity and mortality, and the treatment of choice is insertion of a cardiac pacemaker to prevent severe bradycardia and an anti-arrhythmic drug such as sotalol to suppress the tachycardic episodes.

The value of ambulatory ECG monitoring in old age

There remains some controversy about the value of this method of assessing arrhythmias. Minor

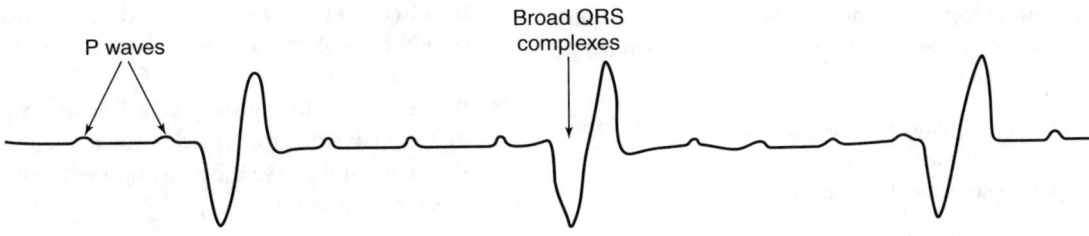

Fig. 13.4 Complete heart block. There is no relationship between P waves and QRS complexes.

arrhythmias are extremely common in old people and the presence of ectopic beats, short runs of tachycardia and short episodes of atrial fibrillation do not correlate well with symptoms. Nevertheless, in patient with blackouts or other symptoms which could be caused by arrhythmias, 24-hour ECG monitoring sometimes uncovers episodes of sustained tachyarrhythmia, sino-atrial bradycardia or the sick sinus syndrome. In such cases, establishing a firm diagnosis can lead to highly beneficial deployment of pacemakers and anti-arrhythmic drugs with very good therapeutic results in a good proportion of the patients.

Important causes of tachyarrhythmias in elderly people

The resting heart rate of a tranquil elderly person should not exceed 100 b.p.m. in health, and sinus tachycardias in response to various stimuli such as exercise or fever are rarely above 130 b.p.m. in people over the age of 75. There are a large number of conditions which can lead to tachyarrhythmias in old people and some of the commoner and more important of these are shown in Box 13.5.

It is important to make a full electrocardiographic diagnosis of the tachyarrhythmia whenever possible, and details of how to go about this can be found in textbooks of cardiology and general medicine. A careful search needs to be made for any underlying predisposing factors, and in the case of a sustained tachyarrhythmia there is a need for urgent treatment to bring the heart rate under control, since the majority of old people will quickly drift into cardiac failure or develop a fatal arrhythmia if left untreated.

Some of the distinguishing features of the different types of tachyarrhythmia are shown in Table 13.1 which illustrates the main differences. The following observations can also be very helpful when differentiating one tachyarrhythmia from another:

- the actual heart rate measured over a full minute, which may be as high as 180 p.m. in a paroxysmal ventricular tachycardia but is

---

Box 13.5 Causes of tachyarrhythmia in old people

Regular tachycardia
- Sinus tachycardia, due to conditions such as fever, cardiac failure, respiratory failure, anaemia, hypovolaemia, adrenergic stimulation, anxiety states, drugs with atropinic or adrenergic properties, thyrotoxicosis
- Supraventricular tachycardias, due to ischaemic heart disease, drug toxicity caused by digoxin and drugs with anticholinergic or adrenergic side-effects, hypokalaemia, anatomical abnormalities in the conducting system etc.
- Ventricular tachycardia, most commonly seen in patients with ischaemic heart disease but can be due to digoxin toxicity or cardiomyopathy; an important complication of myocardial infarction

Irregular tachycardia
- Atrial fibrillation with a poorly controlled ventricular rate; the commonest cause; various predisposing factors described in text
- Sinus tachycardia with frequent ectopic beats; a common cause
- Atrial flutter with varying AV block

---

unlikely to be more than 130 in sinus tachycardia
- the electrocardiographic appearance, and particularly the effect of an intravenous injection of adenosine which blocks AV conduction for a few seconds, and therefore distinguishes a supraventricular tachycardia (SVT) from a ventricular tachycardia (VT)
- the effect on heart rate of carotid sinus massage or other vagotonic manoeuvres, which will often abort an SVT
- the heart rate during sleep which helps to distinguish sinus tachycardia due to anxiety states, in which case the heart rate will fall when the patient is asleep.

Table 13.1   Clinical and electrocardiographic diagnosis of tachycardia.

	Sinus tachycardia	Paroxysmal supra/ventricular tachycardia	Paroxysmal ventricular tachycardia	Atrial flutter	Atrial fibrillation
Usual ventricular rate	120 or less	160–200	150–180	130–160	110–160
Rhythm	Regular	Regular	Regular	Regular	Markedly irregular
Respiratory variation	Yes	None	None	None	None
Minute-to-minute variation	Slight	None	Slight but important	Often quite marked	Marked
Effect of carotid sinus pressure	Slows	Terminates abruptly (and may recur abruptly) or no effect	None	Sudden but transient change	None
Significance	Healthy	Only serious if prolonged; consider K^+ lack or digitalis toxicity	Always serious; requires urgent treatment	Serious; often with organic lesions; may precipitate heart failure	Common accompaniment of organic heart disease; can be 'lone' or with thyrotoxicosis
ECG	P waves present; normal record	Abnormal P waves; QRS normal duration	P waves absent or follow QRS, which is prolonged and deformed	'Saw tooth' regular atrial waves at rate circa 300/min	P waves replaced by irregular, cyclic, atrial waves

Treatment

A detailed account of the treatment of tach-yarrhythmias is outside the scope of this book, but some of the important principles are shown in Box 13.6 (p. 118).

Box 13.6 Some options for treating tachyarrhythmias

- Sinus tachycardia
  - — Diagnose underlying cause and treat.
- Atrial fibrillation
- Atrial flutter
- Supraventricular tachycardia
  - — Convert to sinus rhythm (SR) with direct current (DC) or amiodarone.
  - — Control rate at AV node with digoxin, verapamil or betablockers. Adenosine blocks AV conduction.
  - — prevent recurrence with disopyramide, amiodarone.
- Junctional tachycardia
  - — Try vagal manoeuvres.
  - — Control rate with betablockers, digoxin.
- Ventricular tachycardia
  - — Terminate with lignocaine, betablockers, amiodarone.
  - — DC cardioversion if unstable haemodynamics or no response to drugs.
  - — Prevent with lignocaine, disopyramide, amiodarone.

Alimentary disorders

Introduction

The majority of gastrointestinal illnesses in old people present with the same symptoms as in the young. Furthermore, more or less the same spread of pathology is seen in old age in the gastrointestinal tract, though of course some diseases become commoner with age, particularly gastrointestinal malignancies and diverticular disease. As with pathology in any system, acute gastrointestinal emergencies in frail elderly people sometimes present in an atypical way, with major geriatric problems eclipsing the more typical symptoms. For example, a performated viscus may present with collapse and an acute confusional state, and although physical signs such as tenderness and abdominal rigidity are usually present, they are often less obvious than in the younger person and will only be detected by careful physical examination.

In this chapter we will deal with some aspects of alimentary canal disease which are of particular importance in the practice of geriatric medicine, either because they are common or because they serve to illustrate and emphasize important differences in the mode of presentation in elderly people.

The upper alimentary tract

The mouth and tongue

The tongue has long been regarded as a simple barometer of health and disease and nowhere is this more evident than in old age. It should always, therefore, be examined with care. Almost any systemic illness or illness of the alimentary tract will cause a white or brown furred tongue, a finding which of course is entirely nonspecific. This must be distinguished from oral moniliasis (infection with *Candida albicans*), characterized by white patches not only on the tongue but also on the inner cheeks, gums and fauces (monilial patches are not always easily removable, as food particles are) and the diagnosis can be confirmed by microscopic examination.

Oral candidiasis is a common condition in the elderly and is easily treated with antifungal agents such as fluconazole or nystatin. Smoking, whether pipes or cigarettes, and ill-fitting dentures may also produce tongue changes with a white and sodden appearance of filiform papillae.

A similar appearance can be seen in patients with nicotinic acid deficiency which will improve with supplementation with B-complex vitamins. Nicotinic acid deficiency may produce a red and inflamed-looking tongue. Vitamin B_{12}, folate and iron deficiencies can result in atrophic glossitis. Other important physical signs to note when examining the tongue include the following:

- Fissuring of the tongue and geographical tongue are of no clinical importance.
- Varicosity of the blood vessels on the undersurface of the tongue is due to age changes in the supportive connective tissues.
- A dry tongue is seen in people with inadequate production of saliva, and sometimes in those who persistently mouth-breathe.

- The tongue may be contaminated with food particles in patients with abnormalities of swallowing.
- Hard, indurated areas may be due to carcinoma or premalignant changes such as leukoplakia, and these should be referred immediately to an ear, nose and throat (ENT) specialist.
- The tongue may have a bluish tinge in patients with central cyanosis and may appear pale in those with anaemia.

Dental hygiene

This is important in old people and often neglected. Care should be taken to make sure that dentures fit properly and that natural teeth are in good condition. Patients with carious, loose or painful teeth or severe peridontal disease should be referred to a dentist. Dentures should fit snugly; if they become loose they may require refitting.

However, patients who have been dentureless for many years or have not used dentures will have atrophic gums, in which case it is very difficult to get dentures to fit properly.

Patients with difficulties in chewing or swallowing as a result of cerebrovascular disease or other damage to the bulbar nuclei can only manage dentures if they are very well fitted and held in place with a denture adhesive.

Taste and smell

It is sometimes said that the sensations of taste and smell become less acute with advancing age.

There is some evidence that taste and smell thresholds to some substances rise with age, in which case a higher concentration is required to stimulate the respective nerve endings. However, in the vast majority of elderly people, taste and smell are adequate to enable a person to distinguish food substances, and there seems to be little or no reduction in the pleasure of eating in healthy elderly people.

Acute parotitis

Acute infection of the parotid gland is an important complication of a wide range of severe illnesses in old age. It is caused by ascending infection from the mouth, and is particularly prevalent in patients who are unable to maintain natural oral hygiene because of difficulties with swallowing, mouth breathing or insufficient production of saliva. Occasionally it results from obstruction to the parotid duct by a salivary stone. Treatment is with antibiotics, and it is usually recommended that the antibiotic regimen should include an agent active against anaerobic organisms, such as metronidazole.

In persistent or recurrent parotid infection it is sometimes necessary to perform a sialogram to detect the presence of a stone, or high-resolution ultrasound scan to detect an abscess cavity.

Dysphagia

Dysphagia is a common and very important problem in old age and is usually due to one of the following causes:

- disorders of the nervous control of swallowing
- pressure from outside the oesophagus
- intrinsic disease of the oesophagus.

Neurological causes

As is the case with all other motile viscera of the body, neurological causes of oesophageal dysfunction are important in old age. They may be due to disease within the brain or autonomic nerves or age-related changes in the neuromuscular system. The common neurological disorders in the elderly which lead to dysphagia are stroke, bulbar palsy and presbyoesophagus.

Dysphagia in patients with stroke. Patients with stroke disease can suffer a number of neurological deficits which make swallowing more difficult, and the exact pattern and severity of this will depend on the site of the central nervous system damage.

Therefore, there may be difficulties with sensation in the mouth, tongue and oropharynx, or partial or complete paralysis of the facial muscles, tongue, soft palate and pharynx. Furthermore, the normal coordinated sequencing of swallowing is often lost so patients have difficulty transferring food from the mouth to the oesophagus. In such patients there is a high risk of inhalation of oropharyngeal contents into the lungs, and it is very difficult to maintain natural oral hygiene. In extensive strokes, and particularly if there is bilateral damage in patients with multiple or recurrent stroke, it is often necessary to provide nutrition through a gastrostomy tube, either temporarily or permanently.

Dysphagia due to bulbar palsy. In motor neuron disease and pseudobulbar palsy the difficulty may lie either in transferring the food bolus from the mouth to the oesophagus, or there may be diffuse oesophageal spasm. While these two conditions produce similar effects, they are of quite different aetiology.

Pseudobulbar palsy is associated with bilateral disease of the cerebral cortex, particularly in patients with multi-infarct brain disease, and produces a small spastic tongue and exaggerated jaw jerk. Bulbar palsy due to motor neuron disease affects the bulbar nuclei themselves and produces a wasted fasciculating tongue. Both conditions may produce dysarthria and there are often associated signs of damage in the pyramidal tracts.

As is the case with stroke disease, patients who are experiencing difficulties with swallowing because of bulbar or pseudobulbar palsy can often be helped a great deal from the expert advice of speech therapists, some of whom have a special interest in the management of neurological dysphagia.

Presbyoesophagus

This condition is almost entirely confined to old people and is most commonly seen in the very aged (over 80 years). In this condition the oesophagus becomes poorly coordinated.

There is diffuse oesophageal spasm, and contrast radiology, such as barium swallow, shows abnormalities including loss of coordinated peristalsis, prolonged episodes of oesophageal spasm, and elongation and distortion of the oesophagus to produce the so-called corkscrew oesophagus. Patients with this condition usually learn by trial and error that they can swallow more effectively if they eat soft foods, chew food thoroughly and slow down the speed at which they consume their meal.

Oesophageal spasm can be helped with nitroglycerine. These simple measures will deal with the vast majority of patients, and it is very unusual for the patient to have presbyoesophagus which is so severe that nutrition is compromised.

Obstruction of the oesophagus from without

The oesophagus may be compressed by abnormal enlargement of mediastinal structures. Examples include the following:

- malignant diseases, particularly metastatic deposits in mediastinal lymph nodes
- an aneurysm of the thoracic aorta
- enlargement of the cardiac chambers
- an oesophageal (pharyngeal) pouch, particularly when this is large and filled with food.

Patients with a pharyngeal pouch will also complain of regurgitation of undigested food, often several hours after it has been swallowed.

Dysphagia arising from disease of the oesophagus itself

The possibilities are numerous but in old age the most important pathologies to be considered include:

- carcinoma of the oesophagus, which unfortunately is often well advanced before it causes obstruction
- reflux oesophagus leading to peptic stricture and which may or may not be associated with hiatus hernia
- achalasia of the cardia
- severe inflammation of the lower oesophagus due to candida infection, with mucosal oedema causing the obstruction.

Other causes are relatively rare but would include stricture as a result of swallowing corrosive substances, scleroderma, impaction of a food bolus at the lower end of the oesophagus, an epithelial web at the upper end of the oesophagus in patients with iron deficiency anaemia, and rare tumours of the oesophagus such as fibromata and lyomyomata.

Treatment

Some of the approaches to treatment have been mentioned above, and treatment of the other conditions of the oesophagus is exactly the same in old people as in younger people. Since swallowing is such a basic function for life support, every effort must be made to overcome dysphagia in elderly patients unless it is clearly part of the very last stages of a terminal illness, in which case a palliative approach would be more appropriate.

Hiatus hernia

Hiatus hernia is a common condition in old age. In some people it is associated with a great deal of pain and discomfort, but in others it is often completely asymptomatic. If there is associated reflux oesophagitis it may cause prolonged occult bleeding over many months or a year, leading eventually to an iron deficiency anaemia; there is sometimes rapid bleeding causing haematemesis and melaena, in which case it is usually the site of a peptic ulcer. However, since hiatus hernia is so common in old age (in one series it was reported as being present in 70% of people over the age of 70), symptoms and complications cannot always be attributed to the hiatus hernia alone. This diagnostic problem is very similar to that of colonic diverticulosis and cervical spondylosis, which are common conditions in old age and to which symptoms may be attributed which are in fact due to other causes.

Hiatus hernias may be of three anatomical types:

- A sliding hiatus hernia is the usual type seen in old age; it is associated with reflux oesophagitis. The exact causation is not fully understood but the fibrosis caused by oesophagitis may be one mechanism involved, by causing traction on the cardiac end of the stomach through the diaphragm.
- A para-oesophageal or rolling hiatus hernia occurs no more often in the old than in the young. It is due to a herniation of part of the fundus of the stomach alongside the oesophagus through the diaphragm.
- A mixed hiatus hernia has sliding and para-oesophageal components.

- Other forms of diaphragmatic hernia are relatively rare. An example is the Morgagni hernia in which coils of large bowel herniate into the thorax through a defect in the attachment of the diaphragm to the anterior chest wall; this is rarely of any clinical importance.

Reflux oesophagitis

Although patients with sliding hiatus hernia often have reflux oesophagitis, it is also possible to have symptomatic oesophageal reflux in the absence of a hiatus hernia.

The typical symptoms include burning retrosternal discomfort, which may be worsened when the patient stoops or lies flat, and is often relieved by food, antacids or treatment which reduces gastric acid secretion. The pain is often absent and the patient may present with an iron deficiency anaemia or haemorrhage. Since the condition is largely one of disordered motility, the patients often respond quite well to drugs which speed up gastric emptying, such as cisapride, and the symptoms can be controlled effectively, and the complications relieved, by proton pump inhibitors such as omeprazole or H_2 receptor antagonists such as ranitidine. Patients often benefit from simple mechanical measures such as sleeping with the head of the bed slightly raised, and avoidance of stooping. Surgical treatment is very rarely required in elderly patients with a hiatus hernia since the advent of modern medical therapies.

Age-related changes in gastric secretion

There is an increasing frequency of gastric secretion failure and achlorhydria with advancing age. This is associated with the macroscopic and microscopic changes of atrophic gastritis of the gastric mucosal cells.

There is a dramatic reduction in the number of parietal cells and in many individuals this is associated with an antiparietal cell auto-antibody. Patients with complete achlorhydria and severe atrophic gastritis also fail to produce intrinsic factor and will eventually develop vitamin B_{12} deficiency anaemia.

Peptic ulcer

Peptic ulcer disease is very common in old age. It is an important cause of morbidity and mortality, and delays in the diagnosis are more likely to occur in old people than in the young. However, with modern investigations and treatment the vast majority of peptic ulcers can be detected and treated successfully in elderly people, even when they are rather frail, so there is no excuse for not taking a vigorous approach to the management of this condition.

Some important differentiating features of peptic ulcer in old age can be summarized as follows:

- Although the typical symptoms of epigastric pain and dyspepsia may be present, many old people with peptic ulcers present with nonspecific complaints such as poor appetite, weight loss or the symptoms of anaemia.
- Brisk bleeding from a peptic ulcer will often present with acute geriatric problems such as falls, collapse, acute confusion or incontinence. These symptoms may appear before any haematemesis or melaena.

The causes of peptic ulceration are broadly similar in patients of all age groups, though the following points need to be emphasized:

- Most people, including the elderly, with peptic ulcers do not have overt hypersecretion of gastric acid.
- Many old people use nonsteroidal anti-inflammatory drugs, which are an important cause of gastritis and gastric erosions, and contribute to the formation of gastric and duodenal ulcers.
- Chronic gastric infection by *Helicobacter pylori* is an important aetiological factor.
- Peptic ulceration is more likely to occur in people who smoke or have an excessive alcohol intake.
- Patients with any severe acute medical or surgical illness can develop acute gastric or duodenal ulceration.
- Corticosteroid therapy can contribute to the causation of peptic ulcers.

Investigations

The investigation of choice is upper gastrointestinal endoscopy to examine the oesophagus, stomach and first part of the duodenum. In experienced hands this will almost always confirm the diagnosis, and endoscopy also allows biopsies to be taken of gastric ulcers to rule out malignancy and of the gastric mucosa to detect *Helicobacter pylori* infection.

Treatment

Treatment of peptic ulceration is the same in patients of all ages, though the following points are of particular importance:

- Acute bleeding from a peptic ulcer is a medical emergency requiring the same intervention in elderly people as in the young. It must be borne in mind that the elderly tolerate hypovolaemia less well than younger people, so resuscitation needs to be quicker and more rigorous when the patient is old.
- Perforation of a peptic ulcer is a surgical emergency which will often require operative treatment. However, in very frail old people there is evidence that conservative management with nasogastric suction, intravenous fluids, intravenous ranitidine, antibiotics and pain control may result in a better outcome than a major surgical operation.
- Patients with predisposing factors such as smoking, heavy alcohol intake, corticosteroid therapy or nonsteroidal treatment should have these removed or modified whenever possible.
- Suppression of gastric acid with a proton pump inhibitor or H_2 receptor antagonist will promote healing in almost all patients.
- If *Helicobacter pylori* infection is detected it should be treated with antibiotics.
- Patients with a gastric ulcer should have a follow-up endoscopy after about 8 weeks to check healing and for rebiopsy if the ulcer persists, to rule out malignancy.
- Maintenance treatment, usually with an H_2 receptor antagonist, is often required, unless there was an obvious precipitating cause which can be removed or modified permanently.

Diverticulosis of the upper alimentary canal

As is apparent in other hollow organs, the development of diverticulae in the alimentary canal seems to be an age-related phenomenon. They are found in the oesophagus, duodenum and jejunum. In the duodenum some may be secondary to healed ulcers. In the small bowel they are often multiple, in which case they can be associated with the blind loop syndrome and therefore interfere with the absorption of some nutrients, including vitamin B_{12}.

Pancreatitis

The occurrence of pancreatitis increases with age although it still remains a relatively rare condition. The cause is not always obvious, though in some patients it is associated with cholelithiasis, in which case reflux of bile into the pancreas may be part of the aetiology. In some patients, ischaemia of the pancreas secondary to vascular disease may play a part in the causation. Also, pancreatitis is sometimes seen in patients recovering from accidental hypothermia.

The condition may be less obvious in old people than in the young, though the symptoms of abdominal pain and the sign of abdominal tenderness and rigidity are usually present. The serum amylase will be raised, and the treatment of the condition is along standard lines.

The malabsorption syndrome

Age-related changes in the small bowel mucosa

The villi of the mucosa of the small bowel change their shape as they age, becoming shorter and broader. However, in healthy old people, these changes do not lead to significant malabsorption of nutrients, though the reduced surface area available for absorption will reduce the reserve capacity, and therefore predispose elderly people to the development of frank malabsorption in the presence of pathological conditions.

Some of the disorders of the small intestine which can cause malabsorption, and which are of particular importance in old age are shown in Box 14.1.

Box 14.1 Causes of malabsorption in old people

- Coeliac disease – can occur for the first time in old age, or may have been present life-long
- Bacterial overgrowth – particularly in the presence of diverticulosis of the small bowel
- Dermatitis herpetiformis
- Intestinal resection
- Parasitic infestation – prevalent in tropical regions, but may also be seen in temperate countries if the patient has travelled or lived in an endemic area

---

Symptoms

These include diarrhoea or steatorrhoea, abdominal discomfort or pain, and in severe cases there may be weight loss. Symptoms of specific deficiencies may appear.

Mouth ulcers and angular stomatitis are frequent and patients may experience tetany if they are hypocalcaemic, bone pain from osteomalacia or symptoms of peripheral neuropathy and peripheral oedema.

In old age the disease should be considered in the presence of such complaints, particularly if there is a clear history of steatorrhoea.

Investigations

Absorption tests are now rarely performed since they are cumbersome and nonspecific. In an old person with suspected malabsorption the following should be considered:

- *Estimation of stool fat content and microscopy of stool.* These will detect the presence of undigested meat fibres.
- *Barium meal with small bowel follow-through.* This will detect small bowel diverticulosis, strictures, or anatomical alterations caused by previous surgery. Also, patients with malabsorption often have dilatation of the folds

and a change in the fold pattern which helps to support the diagnosis.

- *Jejunal biopsy*. This will often give diagnostic histological evidence, particularly of coeliac disease.
- *Examination of jejunal secretions*. Taken at the same time as the biopsy. This will often help to detect *Giardia lamblia* infestation.
- *Carbon 14 glycocholic acid breath test*. This is used to detect the presence of bacterial overgrowth in the small intestine, a condition which is

sometimes seen in very frail old people, particularly those who are debilitated, and is a complication of small intestinal diverticulosis and postsurgical blind loops.

Treatment of malabsorption

This will not be dealt with in detail in this chapter. The treatment is the same in old people as in the young and the topic is covered in detail in textbooks of general medicine and gastroenterology.

Important conditions of the large bowel in old age

Bowel habit

Although old people as a group seem to be more aware of their bowel habit than younger people and more concerned about constipation, there is no evidence to suggest that in normal old people bowel habit is different from that in the young. Furthermore, there is some evidence to suggest that older people are no more likely to complain of abdominal symptoms than young adults.

Population surveys among representative portions of the population including the elderly suggest that the normal range of bowel habit in Western Europe and North America lies between three motions a day and three a week in people with no significant pathology and that this is the same in all age groups. Nevertheless, old people take laxatives more often than do the young and this may seem to indicate a propensity to constipation.

Constipation

Though bowel habit is the same in healthy old people as in young adults, constipation is an important accompaniment of debility and, therefore, the problem of constipation in old age requires special consideration. Constipation presenting with paradoxical diarrhoea is also common in old age. In such patients the faecal mass becomes hard and irritates the colonic and rectal mucosa so as to increase mucus secretion, thus allowing fluid stool to bypass the constipating mass. This is an impor-

tant cause of faecal incontinence in frail elderly people, and one which can be treated successfully.

Definition of constipation

Constipation may mean one of two things:

- difficult defaecation, possibly because of hardness of stool, but occurring with the normal regularity
- a change in bowel habit so that defaecation becomes less frequent.

It is important to discover which of these two conditions the patient may be complaining of since each may indicate a different cause. Indeed, it is possible for an old person to have a bowel motion every day and still be constipated, with a large mass of stool remaining in the colon.

Stool consistency

The consistency of the stool is likely to be related to diet and to intestinal transit time, that is, the time taken for material which is swallowed to appear in the stool.

In general, a high-residue diet would be associated with a normal intestinal transit time and easily passed, well-formed stools.

Intestinal transit time

Transit times through the gut can be measured by giving the patient appropriate markers to take by mouth and by noting the period of time that it requires for 80% of the markers to be passed rectally. The most convenient way of doing this is to use small capsules filled with barium and to monitor their presence by radiographs.

In a normal person of any age, 80% of the markers will be cleared within 72 hours. In disabled, and therefore immobile, old people, the period of time taken for 80% of the markers to be passed can be in excess of 7 days. Constipation is a particular menace in immobile old people, partly because physical movement is one of the factors causing the gastrocolic reflex, which is a humoral rather than a neural reflex; entry of food or fluid into the stomach is the other main factor. This reflex is diminished in immobile old people.

In addition, dependence on another person for aid with defaecation may well mean that the need to defaecate occurs when help is not at hand, and the urge may have passed when help is actually given. Constipation is thus one good reason for maintaining mobility; even very minor degrees of exercise such as standing and transferring from chair to bed can be helpful.

Some other important causes of constipation in old age

As people become older many of the factors outlined below become commoner. Furthermore, it is not unusual for an old person to have more than one of these constipating factors present simultaneously. Some important causes of constipation are as follows:

- drugs, particularly opiates, drugs with anticholinergic effects, iron supplements, drugs containing aluminium salts, major tranquillizers
- depression; constipation can be part of the motor retardation of a depressive illness
- carcinoma of the bowel, particularly in the descending colon and rectum
- hypothyroidism
- Parkinson's disease; the constipation in Parkinson's disease is probably due in part to the reduced mobility and in part to parkinsonian autonomic dysfunction
- immobility, as discussed above

- low-residue diet, as discussed above.

The treatment of constipation

The essential step is to make a diagnosis of the cause of the constipation, then to treat the constipation itself and the underlying cause, often with special reference to diet and mobility. In some patients specific interventions will be required: for example, surgery for carcinoma of the colon or thyroxine for hypothyroidism. More often, constipation is the result of immobility and a low-residue diet. Of course, it is not always possible to enable a disabled old person to take regular exercise and in such a person a high-residue diet alone may not relieve the constipation. Therefore, regular treatment in such cases with one treatment or a combination of treatments such as purgatives, suppositories or enemas can be very good medical practice.

The commonly used purgatives are summarized in Box 14.2. However, since these treatments form an important part of geriatric practice a fuller explanation of the mechanism of action of these purgatives is required.

Bulk purgatives. Bulk purgatives take up large amounts of water and this results in a large-volume soft stool. Bran is a natural bulk purgative and can be used to increase the residue of the diet, either by taking bread made with unrefined flour, or by sprinkling powdered bran on the food. Other bulk purgatives include agar and a number of hydrophilic gums, but these should not be used in preference to cereal fibre supplements. Lactulose also acts partly as a bulk purgative by altering intraluminal pH in the colon, which slows down water absorption and leads to a bulkier soft stool.

Lubricant purgatives. Dioctyl sodium sulphosuccinate and poloxalkol reduce the surface tension of faecal matter and thus allow penetration and retention of water in the stool mass. This results in a larger stool volume and a softer stool texture. It is thought that liquid paraffin works partly by changing stool surface tension and partly by a direct softening action, and the term 'lubricant purgative' may in fact be a misnomer since lubrication in the mechanical sense is probably not part of the mode of action. Liquid paraffin, despite its popularity, is not recommended in elderly patients because of the

---

Box 14.2 Classification of the purgatives

Bulk
- Bran
- Agar
- Mucilaginous gums
- Lactulose (altered gut pH causes fluid retention)

Lubricant
- Liquid paraffin
- Dioctyl sodium sulphosuccinate
- Poloxalkol

Irritant
- Senna
- Cascara
- Sodium picosulphate
- Bisacodyl
- Phenolphthalein
- Castor oil

---

risk of inhalation lipid pneumonia, particularly in patients with swallowing difficulty. Furthermore, it can reduce the absorption of fat-soluble vitamins and thereby predispose the patient to osteomalacia.

Irritant purgatives. The third and most widely used group of purgatives in the elderly are the irritant purgatives. There are four main groups in common use: the anthracenes, bisacodyl, sodium picosulphate and phenolphthalein.

The anthracenes include cascara, senna and castor oil. These are absorbed from the small bowel, and broken down in the liver to the active principle emodin which is excreted into the large bowel where it has an irritant effect on the myenteric plexus. The most important member of this group in normal usage is senna, usually prescribed as one of the standardized preparations. Bisacodyl is not absorbed from the gut but has a direct stimulant effect on the myenteric plexus and it may, therefore, be given orally or rectally. Phenolphthalein also has a direct effect on large intestinal smooth muscle.

Suppositories. Bisacodyl and glycerine suppositories are useful in geriatric practice. They are particularly useful when the rectum is distended with a hard or soft stool mass.

Enemas. Large-bulk soap and water enemas are no longer recommended in old people, partly because of the possibility of producing shock as a result of rapid rectal distention, and partly because of the possibility of rupturing a colonic diverticulum. Small-bulk phosphate enemas, however, are very suitable. They contain about 130 ml of hygroscropic substances such as sodium acid phosphate and sodium phosphate. Such phosphate enemas are conveniently presented in disposable packages. Great care must be taken in using these, since there are reports of trauma to the anal canal or rectal mucosa from a nozzle, which can be followed by necrosis, particularly in the presence of a hypertonic solution.

Choice of treatment

The type of treatment depends on the type of constipation. The most severe form of constipation is associated with faecal impaction in which the longstanding presence of faeces in the sigmoid colon and rectum has lead to the development of hard, impacted masses which will, if large enough, require digital breakdown before being passed.

Fortunately, such severe constipation is relatively uncommon. The majority of patients with such severe constipation can be helped by giving a stool-softening agent by mouth followed by a series of low-volume enemas or suppositories.

Irritant purgatives are not recommended in the management of severe faecal impaction because they are likely to result in severe abdominal pain.

In severe constipation, therefore, the objective must be to have the whole rectum and colon emptied by suppositories or enemas, and it must be remembered that this procedure is likely to require the use of these agents for up to 7–10 days to clear the colon properly; securing one evacuation from the lower bowel of a constipated old person is not sufficient as only the rectum is likely to be emptied and further masses of firm or hard faeces will quickly move round from the rest of the colon. Daily treatment is required, therefore, until the enema is returned without any faeces and clinical examination indicates that rectum and colon are empty. Extensive constipation which falls short of actual faecal impaction will respond to similar treatment, though in such cases there is often an equally good result from use of an irritant laxative, and picosulphate preparations have been particularly helpful in this context.

Once constipation has been completely dealt with, the need to prevent its recurrence must be considered. If the constipation has resulted from the patient's immobility and if the immobility remains, then some additional treatment is needed.

This may be the use of a combined stool softener and anthracene purgative, or in some patients it may be necessary to give regular suppositories or low-volume enemas once or twice a week. Sometimes a combined approach is required, and the most appropriate treatment, its frequency and dosage will vary from individual to individual. The advantage of a small enema or of suppositories is that a result is obtained within a short period of time and the attendant can be sure of their effectiveness. A disadvantage is that they are usually required to be given by a nurse. The irritant purgatives on the other hand have the disadvantage that they can cause faecal incontinence in old people. There have been reports of degeneration of Auerbach's plexus as a result of the long-term regular use of anthracene purgatives, but there is no conclusive evidence that this is of clinical importance in elderly people.

Megacolon

Idiopathic megacolon occurs more commonly among old people than among the young and also more commonly among immobile and institutionalized populations than among those at home. There are probably several factors involved in its production. These are:

- immobility leading to longstanding constipation
- the long-term use of anticholinergic drugs
- a possible effect due to age-related changes in the peripheral autonomic plexuses.

Idiopathic megacolon often presents with faecal incontinence and may be suspected from the considerable distention of the abdomen with gas. It is not an easy condition to treat. The first approach is usually the treatment of constipation as outlined above, and some clinicians have advocated the use of cholinergic drugs such as bethanechol. Idiopathic megacolon occasionally leads to intestinal obstruction due to severe constipation, or volvulus of the sigmoid colon.

Sometimes a volvulus will be corrected by sigmoidoscopy with insufflation of the large bowel, but over 50% of cases require operative surgical treatment.

Other diseases of the colon which are important in the elderly

Diverticular disease

The development of colonic diverticula becomes more common with increasing age. They are almost never found in the young but in Western Europe and North America the prevalence rises steadily above the age of 50, and in some surveys it reaches as high as 40% of people over the age of 80. There is some evidence, though this is not conclusive, that a change back to a more fibrous diet in some sections of the European and North American population is leading to a fall in the prevalence of diverticular disease. The development of colonic diverticula with age is not found in parts of the world where a high-residue diet is taken by the majority of the population, so the disease is rare in most parts of Africa, South and South-east Asia and South America.

Further evidence which relates colonic diverticulosis to a low-residue diet is the fact that during the Second World War, when bread was produced with unrefined flour in Great Britain, the incidence of diverticulitis dropped and that, by contrast, the disease was only reported with any frequency from the beginning of the 20th century when widespread use of refined flour became common. Finally, it has been shown that rats fed on a low-residue diet develop colonic diverticula whereas those on a normal-residue diet do not.

The clinical significance of colonic diverticula

Since colonic diverticula commonly develop as an accompaniment of ageing, great caution must be observed in attributing to diverticular disease the development of bowel symptoms. The demonstration of diverticulosis on a barium enema is not in itself sufficient evidence in old people that their symptoms are due to this cause. Therefore, care must be taken to exclude other possible causes of symptoms.

The pathogenesis of colonic diverticulosis

The reason why low-residue diets should predispose to the development of diverticulosis has been explained as follows.

At the recto-sigmoid junction there is a functional sphincter which results from the contraction of the transverse muscles of the colon forming the normal colonic haustrations. The areas between haustrations have been compared to bladders by some researchers and the greater the quantity of transverse muscle contraction, the higher the pressure within the bladder. Since this area acts as a functional sphincter, then the less bulky the colonic contents, the greater the frequency of contractions required to prevent the onward passage of faeces to the rectum. On the other hand, the more bulky the faeces, the less contraction needed. Thus in patients on a high-residue diet there is likely to be less high pressure within the colonic bladders and so less likelihood of diverticulosis developing. This principle is illustrated in Figure 14.1.

Another important factor is the strength of the colon wall itself. Diverticula develop between the colonic taenia, particularly at the weak spot where

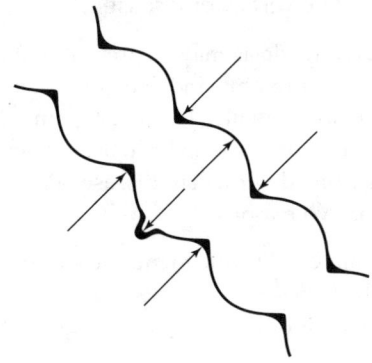

Fig. 14.1 'Bladdering' in the sigmoid colon resulting in colonic diverticulum.

the perforating arteries pass through the colonic wall (see Fig. 14.2).

It is likely that the strength of the colonic wall is impaired with advancing age because of diminished elasticity within the connective tissues, and this together with the increased pressure within the segments of the colon leads to the development of diverticula.

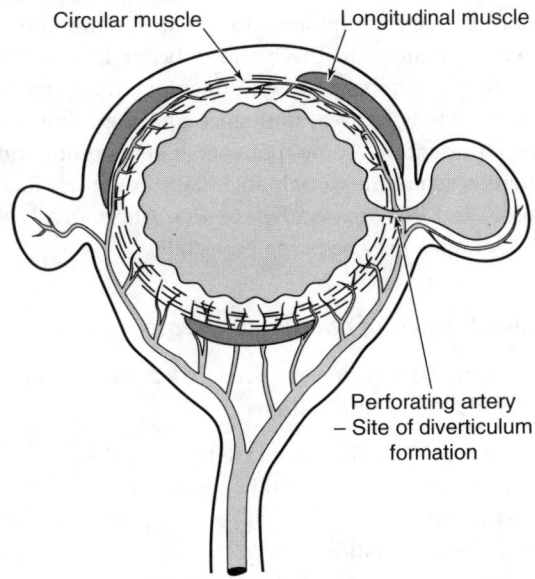

Fig. 14.2 Cross-section of the colon indicating diverticulum formation.

Symptoms of diverticular disease

Colonic diverticulosis may be present without producing any symptoms and the condition may be discovered incidentally. However, pain occurs in about 80% of patients who have been diagnosed as suffering from diverticular disease. Pain may be present for two reasons:

- as a result of colic due to muscle spasm as described above
- as a result of inflammation.

The pain itself is not diagnostic of diverticulosis and it may often be relieved by antispasmodic treatment such as the anticholinergic drug propantheline. Pain and tenderness in the left iliac fossa are often found in patients with diverticular disease.

Change in bowel habit is another important symptom and this may be the development of either diarrhoea or constipation, though the latter is the more common. Some patients develop alternating constipation and diarrhoea.

The third important symptom is rectal bleeding which occurs in about 30% of patients in whom a diagnosis of diverticular disease has been made. The close relationship of the perforating artery to the diverticulum explains why bleeding is so common. Urinary symptoms, due to an inflammatory area contiguous to the bladder, occur in a small number of patients. Other alimentary tract symptoms such as nausea, flatulence and vomiting are also present in some patients. On examination there is sometimes a palpable mass in the left iliac fossa, and this area is often tender. Alternatively a tender mass may be palpated rectally.

Complications of diverticular disease

These are largely due to infection, leading to one of the following complications:

- diverticulitis, in which case there is infection with inflammation within one or more diverticula
- abscess formation
- formation of a fistula from a diverticular abscess into the bladder, vagina or another part of the alimentary tract

- perforation, which may lead to peritonitis
- extensive fibrosis, which can occur around inflamed diverticular disease and cause a stricture leading to intestinal obstruction.

In all but the most acute cases, treatment involves a high-residue diet and the use of antispasmodic drugs. In severe acute cases of diverticulitis it may be necessary to give temporarily a fluid diet and pethidine to control symptoms.

Morphine should be avoided as this will increase the colonic motility and aggravate the underlying causative mechanism. Active diverticulitis will require treatment with antibiotics and it is occasionally necessary to perform a surgical operation for some of the complications of diverticulitis.

Carcinoma of the colon and rectum

Cancer of the alimentary tract is one of the commonest causes of death in old age, and excluding the prostate, the alimentary tract is the commonest site of malignant disease. If there is any change in bowel habit, carcinoma of the colon and rectum must be considered. If carcinoma is suspected and cannot be diagnosed by rectal examination, a sigmoidoscopy must be carried out and followed by investigation of the entire colon.

There are three main methods of investigating the colon, each with certain advantages and disadvantages as follows:

- *Colonoscopy.* Fibreoptic colonoscopy allows the entire colon and the last few centimetres of the small bowel to be inspected visually. The main advantage is that, in skilled hands, very few malignant tumours will be missed. Colonoscopy also gives the opportunity to take biopsy samples, remove polyps, assess gastrointestinal motility and see mucosal lesions such as angiodysplasia. The main disadvantage is that a very thorough preparation of the colon is required, including purgatives which frail people find very tiring. The procedure itself is also fairly uncomfortable.
- *Standard double-contrast barium enema.* This is a tried and tested method which at its best will

give very few false negative results. The main advantages are that permanent records can be obtained, and serious pathologies are unlikely to be missed.

Disadvantages include a fairly arduous purgative preparation, the discomfort of the procedure, the inability to take biopsy specimens and the possibility that rectal disease will be missed.

- *Computed tomography (CT) scan with barium contrast.* This technique has gained favour in investigating frail elderly patients. Although the accuracy of the technique is rather less than standard double-contrast barium enema and colonoscopy, the main advantage is that much less preparation is required. Another advantage is that other intra-abdominal structures can be scanned and assessed at the same time.

Abdominal ultrasound scanning can also be helpful to confirm the presence of a mass. It is sometimes argued that investigations of these types are expensive and disagreeable and should not be used in old age to make the diagnosis of malignant disease if surgery is not going to be used.

While there are occasions when the argument is appropriate, in general it is essential to establish a diagnosis at any age since treatable conditions may always be found and in any case the management of terminal malignant disease can be embarked on with much more confidence if the diagnosis is certain.

Furthermore, the surgical cure rate for carcinoma of the colon without lymph node involvement is now very good at all ages, with 5-year survival rates in some series as high as 80% Modern surgical techniques also allow most resections to be performed, even in the rectum, as a one-stage operation without colostomy.

Ischaemic colitis

Since one of the features of old age is the development of arteriosclerotic vascular disease, it might be anticipated that ischaemic colitis will be a condition as common as transient cerebral ischaemia and ischaemic heart disease.

However, this is not the case and the reason for this is probably the nature of the blood supply to the large bowel. This is shown in Figure 14.3, where it may be clearly seen that the two major blood vessels, the superior mesenteric and inferior mesenteric arteries, divide first into a number of major branches and that these in turn supply the gut through a series of arcades which are all linked together by a marginal artery.

The marginal artery thus provides a major anastomotic channel and for this reason minor degrees of ischaemia in the colon are relatively uncommon, although major gangrene due to obstruction of the superior or inferior mesenteric arteries themselves is an occasional surgical emergency in the elderly. Ischaemic colitis, however, does occur and must always be suspected in a patient presenting with the following symptoms:

- episodes of abdominal pain
- blood-stained diarrhoea.

The most vulnerable area of the colon is the splenic flexure, the watershed between the two major arteries. Attacks of ischaemic colitis may occur with

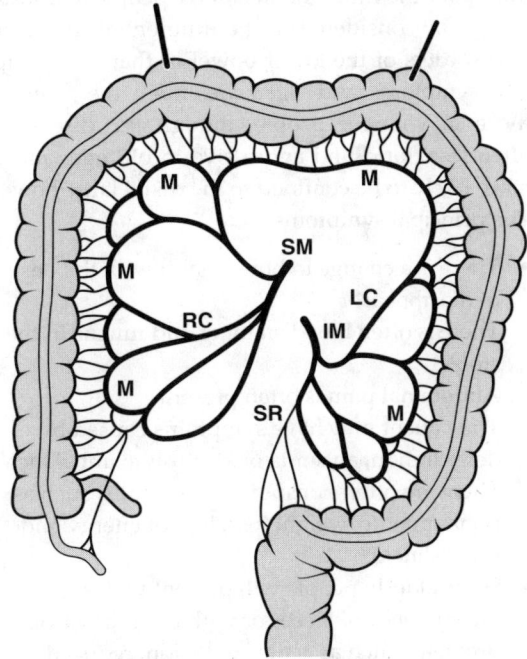

Fig. 14.3 Blood supply to the colon. SM = superior mesenteric; IM = inferior mesenteric; RC = right colic; LC = left colic; SR = superior rectal; M = marginal.

no apparent warning though one of the following predisposing factors is often present.

- a drop in blood pressure
- hypovolaemia or dehydration
- congestive cardiac failure.

The condition usually occurs suddenly and may be associated with an intense fear of food. Abdominal pain and loose stools containing red blood or blood clot confirm the suspicion and a diagnosis can be made definitely by barium enema.

Ischaemic colitis is transitory since tissue infarction is unlikely to occur, though there is inflammatory oedema and exudate which may be followed much later by a degree of fibrous tissue scarring.

Therefore, a barium enema performed at the time of the acute illness shows an area of oedema, which is sometimes likened to thumb imprints, and the same investigation performed at a later date may show a stricture.

Ischaemic colitis is treated expectantly with a fluid diet and if analgesics are required then pethidine should be used. Hypotension must be managed, and any concomitant congestive cardiac failure or other coexisting conditions require optimal management.

Mesenteric artery occlusion on the other hand, leads to infarction and gangrene of a large bowel segment. This is a surgical emergency which requires early operative treatment and carries a substantial mortality rate.

Inflammatory bowel disease in elderly people

Ulcerative colitis

Ulcerative colitis is known to occur quite commonly for the first time in elderly people and must always be considered in the differential diagnosis of disorders of the lower bowel in that age group. The symptoms and signs are much the same as those in younger people, though the disease is often less florid and aggressive in old age, and is more likely to be confined to the distal large bowel. The principal symptoms are:

- There is a change in bowel habit with the onset of diarrhoea.
- There is often blood staining and mucus in the stool.
- Abdominal pain is often present.
- The patient may have symptoms caused by dehydration, anaemia or electrolyte imbalance.
- There are often nonspecific symptoms such as poor appetite, weight loss, loss of energy and feverishness.
- Some elderly people will present with incontinence of faeces or with other geriatric problems such as acute confusion, reduced mobility and failure to cope, particularly if they have become very dehydrated or anaemic.

The most commonly found physical signs are:

- There is abdominal tenderness, which may be generalized, or in patients with distal colitis may be confined to the left iliac fossa.
- There is often abdominal distention which may be severe in a patient with toxic megacolon.
- Severe tenderness and absence of bowel sounds is suggestive of perforation of the bowel with peritonitis.
- Patients with an acute attack of ulcerative colitis are usually slightly tachycardic and often have a slightly low blood pressure and mild fever.

The diagnosis and management of the condition is the same in old age as in younger people. Similarly, the indications for surgical intervention are the same in old age and will not be reiterated in detail in this chapter.

Long-term maintenance with drugs such as olsalazine and mesalazine, and sometimes maintenance steroid treatment, will keep the disease process under reasonable control in the majority of patients.

Distal proctitis

A less severe form of ulcerative colitis, sometimes known as granular proctitis, presents as diarrhoea or faecal incontinence in old age. It is not associated with blood in the stool and sigmoidoscopy shows a uniform hyperaemic velvety appearance of the rectal mucosa. This condition is usually treated very successfully by a series of hydrocortisone hemisuccinate enemas, and maintenance therapy with olsalazine keeps the disease process under control in the majority of patients.

Crohn's disease

This is often thought of as a disease of young adults, but a second peak in the incidence occurs in those over the age of 70. Crohn's disease in the old is the only one of the colonic diseases likely also to affect the anus. Barium enema may show the typical string sign, indicating involvement of discrete localized areas.

In some old people Crohn's disease will present with predominantly geriatric problems such as faecal incontinence, debility and failure to cope, though the presence of abdominal pain and diarrhoea should alert the clinician to the possibility of intra-abdominal disease which will then lead eventually to an appropriate diagnosis.

Treatment is along the same lines as in younger adults.

Intestinal angiodysplasia

Angiodysplasia, characterized by areas of fragile new vessel formation in the submucosal layer of the gastrointestinal tract, has become recognized as an important source of acute and chronic haemorrhage.

These areas occur throughout the gastrointestinal tract, though they are probably commoner in the colon and in that site are generally more accessible to treatment. They increase with advancing age and are most likely to present with episodes of unexplained gastrointestinal haemorrhage or iron deficiency anaemia. They cannot be detected by barium contrast radiography, CT scanning or ultrasound.

They are sometimes visible on colonoscopy, and in very difficult diagnostic cases can be detected by angiography if they are bleeding or extensive. Small, frequently bleeding segments of angiodysplasia sometimes require surgical resection, though in many cases colonic angiodysplasia can be treated by cauterization via colonoscopy.

Electrolyte and body fluid disorders

Changes in electrolyte and water homeostasis with advancing age

Advancing age does not bring any fundamental change in water and electrolyte homeostasis, though it does bring a reduced capacity of the homeostatic responses necessary when steady state conditions are perturbed by pathology or extreme conditions.

The most important of the organs involved, the kidney, loses functional ability steadily throughout life. The mean glomerular filtration rate (GFR) corrected to a standardized surface area falls by about 40% between the ages of 30 and 80. There is also an age-related decline in renal concentrating activity which is independent of the fall in GFR. Another organ involved, particularly in acid-base homeostasis, is the lung, which shows progressive loss of function as age advances, and its compensatory powers also become limited, though in the absence of overt lung pathology, pulmonary reserve is sufficient to cope with most metabolic circumstances.

The importance of electrolyte and body fluid disorders in geriatric practice

Physicians dealing with elderly patients encounter a large number of people with disturbed electrolyte and fluid balance. The fundamental mechanisms leading to such disturbances are the same in patients of any age and are dealt with in great detail in textbooks of metabolic and general medicine. In this chapter we will concentrate on a number of issues within this greater topic which are of particular importance in the general medical care of elderly people. These are:

- water depletion
- low sodium syndromes
- potassium depletion
- potassium excess.

Water depletion

The term water depletion is used in preference to dehydration, which is often loosely used to mean either a pure water loss or loss of salt and water together; these two conditions have different causes and require different management so it is important to use the terms accurately.

In health the total body water is kept constant over an appreciable period of time by adjusting the amount of liquid drunk to equal the losses in urine, breath and sweat. The fluid input is controlled by thirst, a sensation known to all.

The slaking of thirst is an activity taken for granted by healthy alert adults; we feel thirst, we know what the sensation means, we take steps to remove it by getting fluid ourselves (or getting others to do it for us) and then we drink. Though normal people slake their thirst more or less unthinkingly, the water balance of ill, old people is often jeopardized because they fail in one or more of the four steps mentioned above. Thus:

- Thirst sensation can be blunted. As people age

the osmostat responsible for detecting a rise in blood osmolality is less sensitive, which causes the sensation of thirst to be experienced later and less intensely than in younger people. There is also evidence that people with central nervous system diseases such as vascular dementia can have an even less efficient thirst mechanism.

- Although the patient is aware of the thirst sensation, there is recognition neither of its meaning nor of the action required. This will occur in people with central nervous system damage due to cerebral infarction, vascular dementia, Alzheimer's disease and other diffuse brain disorders leading to cognitive decline. Even when the perception of thirst sensation is intact, and its significance and the action required are understood, fluid may not be accessible because action is impeded by immobility due to apathy, stupor or physical limitation of movement.
- When all other mechanisms are intact, including perception of thirst, correct biological response and access to fluid, there may be mechanical difficulties with swallowing which makes fluid intake very restricted or impossible.

The patients most at risk of water depletion are the mentally confused, those in coma or stupor, and those with a fever. Water depletion itself can cause mental disturbances and will tend to make existing confusion worse.

Water depletion often goes unrecognized.

The sufferers may be unable to express their needs, and the signs of water lack are inconspicuous, but, like all diagnoses, water depletion is easy to recognize, and to correct, once the possibility is considered.

It is important to keep water lack in mind in any old person who has been:

- comatose or stuporous for more than 24 hours
- immobilized in isolation for any reason
- demented or confused with breakdown of social organization
- febrile
- suffering from vomiting and/or diarrhoea (in which case there will be electrolyte loss also).

The physical signs of water depletion are unimpressive until the condition is severe. The skin is dry, but does not have the same lack of turgor that characterizes loss of both salt and water. Likewise, the tongue is dry and often furred because the patient is lethargic and not eating, and is not able to keep the mouth clean. Usually, the blood pressure does not fall, nor is there venous collapse as is seen in salt depletion, until the patient is severely water-depleted.

Confirmation of the diagnosis of water depletion is simply obtained: a venous blood sample will usually show increased concentrations of the serum electrolyte values. For example, in moderately severe water depletion the following values will be typical:

- Serum sodium is raised into the range of 155–160 mmol/l (normal range 135–145).
- Serum potassium level is usually in the range of 5–6 mmol/l (normal range 3.6–5.2).
- Blood urea will have risen above the normal range.
- The rate of urine flow is low, and the urine is highly coloured and has a high specific gravity.
- Serum osmalality will be raised above the normal range (285–295 mosmol/kg)

Treatment

Treatment is relatively straightforward:

- free access to water and encouragement to drink in those who are mentally clear and not physically prevented from drinking
- free, easy access to water and supervision as to ensure adequate drinking actually occurs in the confused
- infusions of isotonic dextrose intravenously in those who are stuporous, comatose or physically prevented from drinking.

The total amount of fluid needed for replacement can be roughly gauged from the following formula:

$$Vol(1) = \frac{(serum\ Na\ mmol/l - 140 \times body\ weight\ (kg))}{200}$$

For example, a 50 kg patient with serum sodium of 156 mmol/l would require 4 litres of fluid. Once the water deficit has been made up, conscious patients will automatically regulate their own fluid intake.

Low sodium syndromes

A common problem in frail elderly patients is the finding of a low serum sodium concentration. The reference range, based on studies in healthy old people, is 135–145 mmol/l, and values of 132 or less qualify as definite hyponatraemia. Some of the common and important causes of hyponatraemia in old people are shown in Box 15.1.

Box 15.1 Common causes of hyponatraemia

- True sodium depletion
- The quartet of a low serum sodium concentration, oedema resistant to diuretics, persistent congestive heart failure and pre-renal uraemia
- Iatrogenic water excess ⎫
- Excessive antidiuretic hormone effect from certain neoplasms ⎬ Causing 'dilutional' hyponatraemia
- Hyponatraemia of unknown mechanism occurring in the course of severe general disease

---

The two commonest causes are true sodium depletion and a low sodium concentration in the context of persistent congestive heart failure, diuretic therapy and pre-renal uraemia.

True sodium depletion

By true sodium depletion is meant a state in which the total sodium content of the body has fallen.

Loss of sodium inevitably entails some water loss, the brunt of which falls on the extracellular fluid (ECF) and plasma with relatively little change in intracellular fluid (ICF) volume. The clinical signs are dominated by four factors:

- reduced turgor of the subcutaneous tissues due to depletion of interstitial fluid

- the circulatory effects of reduction in plasma volume
- the intrinsic water intoxication effects of a low serum sodium concentration
- attendant disturbances in acid-base balance.

Loss of tissue turgor gives rise to a gaunt, desiccated general appearance. The eyes are sunken and eyeball tension is low. Dryness and furring of the tongue and lips make speech and chewing difficult. The skin is lank, and when a fold on the limbs or abdomen is pinched up between the examiner's fingers, it remains deformed for longer than normal.

Circulatory examination reveals collapsed jugular veins and the signs of reduced cardiac output. Peripheral pulses are of small volume and the blood pressure is low, often with a large orthostatic fall. In more advanced sodium lack, with gross reduction of blood volume, there is intense peripheral vasoconstriction with cold, cyanotic extremities and a very low blood pressure.

Causes of true sodium depletion

The causes of sodium depletion in old people are much the same as in younger adults. Common ones include:

- *Loss of upper intestinal secretions.* This will occur, for example, in small bowel obstruction with vomiting, therapeutic aspiration of small bowel contents and in the presence of fistulae between the small and large bowel, and can occur in patients with a jejunostomy or ileostomy.
- *Severe watery diarrhoea.* The typical cause will be acute gastroenteritis, usually due to viral or bacterial infection. The most florid examples will be seen in the specific acute bacterial infections such as severe *Salmonella* gastroenteritis, infection with enteropathogenic or enterotoxigenic *E. coli*, bacillary dysentery and cholera.
- *Iatrogenic diarrhoea.* An important cause is enterocolitis due to rapid overgrowth of *Clostridium difficile* in patients who have been

treated with broad-spectrum antibiotics. This can occur after almost any antibiotic which suppresses the normal flora, though particular problems have been experienced with cephalosporins, broad-spectrum penicillins and ciprofloxacin. The condition can occur in patients treated either orally or intravenously. The diarrhoea can be severe.

- *Excessive treatment with laxatives or magnesium sulphate.*
- *Excessive diuresis in patients treated with powerful diuretics.*
- *Severe therapeutic dietary sodium restriction.*
- *Renal loss of sodium.* This takes place in conditions such as chronic salt-losing nephropathy or patients who have had sudden relief of chronic urinary obstruction, or in the recovery phase from acute nephritis.
- *Osmotic diuresis.* An example is that occurring in diabetic coma.

Persistent low sodium concentrations in patients with congestive heart failure

This is a very common set of circumstances in old people. It is not infrequent to see a persistently low serum sodium level in people with chronic congestive cardiac failure requiring long-term treatment with potent diuretics.

In this state, although the serum sodium concentration is often greatly lowered, the patient's cardiac failure often gradually worsens and the physical signs of congestive cardiac failure persist with a raised jugular venous pressure, intractable peripheral oedema and engorgement of the liver. The serum sodium may be depressed even further in patients who are being simultaneously treated with an angiotensin converting enzyme inhibitor. Emergence of this clinical picture signifies the late stages of chronic heart failure.

The sensible approach under these circumstances is to get good symptomatic control of the cardiac failure, to avoid using excessive amounts of diuretic if possible and to accept that the patient may remain chronically hyponatraemic. Under these circumstances, the patient has a truly reduced body sodium, so water restriction is unlikely to have much effect on the serum sodium value and

may lead to a serious reduction of the circulating blood volume.

Iatrogenic water excess

In this condition there is no loss of sodium from the body, but excess water is introduced, usually in the course of misconceived or ill-controlled parenteral therapy. Water intoxication is only likely to occur when nonsaline fluids are being given either i.v., or by rectal or subcutaneous infusion. In postoperative patients an additional factor is the reduction of urine flow caused by antidiuretic hormone (ADH) secreted in response to pain or opiates.

The symptoms of water excess are:

- mental confusion
- malaise and a feeling of ill health
- headache
- nausea and anorexia.

The physical signs are:

- puffiness of the face and some times generalized oedema
- if there is severe volume overload, a raised jugular venous pressure
- neuromuscular twitching and frank convulsions; these may be fatal.

The condition can be avoided by frequent measurement of the serum sodium concentration and haematocrit in all patients receiving infusions other than normal saline, though the most important factor of all is to base intravenous fluid replacement therapy on a careful assessment of the patient's salt and water requirements, to calculate the volume required as accurately as possible and to control and monitor the volume and rate of the infusion.

When signs of water intoxication have actually appeared, the infusion must be stopped; then if urine flow is rapid and the hyponatraemia is mild, the condition will almost always correct itself. In very severe cases where there may be, for example, convulsions, hypertonic saline solutions can be given, though this must be done very carefully with frequent measurement of the serum sodium concentration and due care to avoid overloading the patient with sodium.

Syndrome of inappropriate secretion of antidiuretic hormone (SIADH)

A number of pathological states can give rise to excess production of antidiuretic hormone. Under these circumstances water is retained at renal level and a dilutional hyponatraemia occurs. The important findings for the diagnosis are:

- a low serum sodium with low serum osmalality
- a simultaneously high urine osmalality
- the detection of antidiuretic hormone in peripheral blood despite a low serum osmalality.

A wide variety of conditions can cause inappropriate antidiuretic hormone secretion and these include some conditions which are common in old age (Box 15.2).

Box 15.2 Some important causes of inappropriate ADH secretion

- **Neoplasms**
  - Carcinoma of the bronchus is the most likely neoplasm to be implicated, though the syndrome can be seen with other tumours in the thorax and upper gastrointestinal tract, e.g. carcinoma of the oesophagus, carcinoma of the pancreas.

- **Infections**
  - Particularly pneumonia and septicaemia but the condition can also be seen in tuberculosis and a variety of other focal and generalized infections.

- **Head injury**
  - Intracranial bleeding leading to subdural or extradural haematoma or cerebral haemorrhage.

- **Stroke**
- **Hypothyroidism**
- **Positive pressure ventilation**
- Various drugs including thiazide, diuretics, narcotic agonists and tricyclic antidepressants.
- Emotional distress is probably also another precipitating cause.

The clinical features of inappropriate ADH secretion

These are very similar to those which can be seen in patients with iatrogenic water excess (see above).

Patients who have developed inappropriate ADH secretion gradually often have relatively few symptoms other than lethargy and a poor appetite, but when intense ADH secretion is causing a rapid fall in the serum sodium, the patients are often very weak, complain of headache and poor concentration, and may develop neuromuscular twitching or convulsions.

Hyponatraemia of uncertain cause

In a proportion of patients with hyponatraemia, no clearly defined cause will be found. Some presumably have what have been described as new steady states; that is, they respond normally to changes of salt intake and their condition is not improved by hypertonic saline. Others, at the end of their lives, can have a generalized breakdown of the mechanisms in cell membranes which maintain the electrolyte pattern of intracellular fluid against a concentration gradient. Yet others possibly entail a disturbance of the set point of the osmotic receptors in the hypothalamus. In patients who fall into this broad category, once the treatable causes of hyponatraemia have been excluded, there is no need for further investigation and intervention, particularly if the patient is in a clinically stable condition and relatively asymptomatic.

Potassium depletion

Deficiency of potassium is a common and important disorder in old people: common because many conditions lead to a deficiency of potassium, and important because the effects are serious and sometimes lethal, but often correctable.

The physiological effects of potassium depletion

Potassium is the main cation of intracellular fluid where it is present in concentrations of about 100 mmol/1. Its presence influences many enzymes reactions, so depletion of potassium below the optimal level causes severe functional disturbances; if the deficiency is prolonged and profound, irreversible organic changes eventually occur.

About 70% of the body's potassium is inside skeletal muscle cells, so it is not surprising that the main brunt of potassium deficiency falls on muscle; cardiac and intestinal smooth muscle are also affected.

The causes of potassium deficiency

Some common causes of potassium depletion are listed as single items in Box 15.3 but it is important to remember that several different causes may be operating simultaneously to produce potassium depletion, and also that a deficiency of potassium is often merely one aspect of a complicated metabolic illness.

Inadequate dietary intake.   Young adults take, on average, between 50 and 150 mmol of potassium daily in their diet. Most old people have a potassium intake which is right at the lower end of this range and many teeter perpetually on the brink of potassium lack. Some degree of depletion is probably inevitable if the daily intake of potassium falls below 25 –35 mmol per day. A purely dietary deficiency develops slowly and is rarely the cause of severe symptoms; usually nothing more than mild impairment of muscular strength and general lethargy results, but this low-key potassium deficiency can set the scene for an unexpectedly severe effect when potassium loss results from some acute disturbance such as diarrhoea or accidental trauma.

Box 15.3 Some common causes of potassium depletion

- Inadequate dietary intake
  - poor diet
  - isolation
  - poverty
  - apathy
  - severe loss of appetite
- Diuretic therapy
- Steroid therapy
- Diarrhoea
  - Abuse of purgatives
  - Ulcerative colitis
  - Severe diverticulitis
  - Steatorrhoea
  - Villous papilloma of the colon
  - Severe gastrointestinal infection
- Trauma
  - Severe tissue injury or anoxia
  - Fracture
  - Surgical operation
- Loss of intestinal secretions
  - Aspiration of intestinal contents
  - Fistulae
  - Vomiting

Most of the obligatory daily potassium loss is renal, though about 5–10 mmol of potassium is lost per day in the stool. These losses are inevitable and continue even when potassium depletion is severe.

Diuretics.   Cardiac failure is very common in old people and diuretic therapy still forms the cornerstone of treatment. Consequently, diuretics are now the chief offenders in causing a low serum potassium concentration, though it must be emphasized that the majority of patients taking a diuretic for cardiac failure do not have low serum potassium concentrations, and the majority have whole body potassium contents within the normal range. There is no sound evidence to support the practice of routinely giving potassium supplements to patients taking an oral diuretic; patients given potassium are as likely to develop hypokalaemia as those taking a diuretic alone. However, serum potassium levels should be monitored, particularly in the early stages of diuretic therapy, and it is advisable to give potassium supplements to patients whose serum potassium falls below 3 mmol/l.

The use of combination diuretics containing so-called potassium-sparing drugs are of little benefit and are particularly prone to cause hyponatraemia in elderly subjects.

Diarrhoea. Potassium depletion can result not only from profuse watery diarrhoea, as, for example, in acute gastroenteritis, but also from the passage of frequent, bulky but formed stools as in severe steatorrhoea.

Many old people believe that it is essential to have at least one motion per day, and thereby develop the habit of taking excessive amounts of anthracene and phenolphthalein laxatives. These drugs are potent causes of potassium loss in the stool and can cause insidious, though very severe, potassium depletion. Inflammatory bowel disease, particularly ulcerative colitis, when in relapse can cause fulminant potassium deficiency which can be life-threatening.

Tissue trauma or anoxia. Oxygen lack or trauma to tissues, especially to skeletal muscle, causes potassium to move out of cells into the ECF. In the early stages this will merely cause a slightly elevated serum potassium concentration, but because the quantity of potassium filtered at the glomerulus increases, excretion in the urine rises and a depletion of the electrolyte eventually develops.

Surgical operations, especially when performed on an old person who is already on the edge of potassium deficiency, are a frequent cause of sudden potassium depletion with a brisk drop in the serum potassium concentration.

Symptoms and signs of potassium depletion

Experimentally induced depletion of potassium has shown that depletion up to about 10% of the body total – that is, a loss of about 250 mmol in an old person — will cause no symptoms.

At this level, and with more severe depletion, a fall of the serum potassium concentration occurs only if the sodium intake is simultaneously high. It is of practical importance to realize that under some circumstances, quite severe potassium depletion can exist without the serum potassium concentration being unequivocally low. The symptoms and signs of potassium deficiency, all, some or none of which can be present at any given serum potassium level, are:

- *Muscle weakness.* This is often detectable in ill patients simply as severe generalized lethargy or weakness of the hand grip. In more severe states of potassium depletion, particular muscle groups can show virtually complete paralysis.
- *Mental confusion.*
- *Cardiac arrhythmias and ECG changes.* The electrocardiographic signs of potassium deficiency are important for confirmation of clinical suspicion of potassium depletion, and as a warning that arrhythmias may occur. The ECG signs of hypokalaemia, in order of their evolution, are:
  — flattening of precordial T waves with prolongation of the QT interval
  — the appearance of large U waves
  — sagging of the ST segments
  — fusion of the T and U waves.

These changes are illustrated in Figure 15.1. The changes are reasonably well correlated with the serum potassium value and they are an indication of liability of the appearance of an arrhythmia, which is always a serious event in an old person, and can be fatal.

The most usual arrhythmia is paroxysmal atrial tachycardia with variable atrioventricular block, which may proceed to complete heart block. The most important complication of such an arrhythmia will be the emergence of heart failure in an old person with a sustained tachycardia.

The biochemical findings in potassium depletion

The normal range for serum potassium concentration is 3.6–5.2 mmol/l in elderly people who are well. Values in the range of 2.0–3.5 are commonly seen in severe potassium depletion,

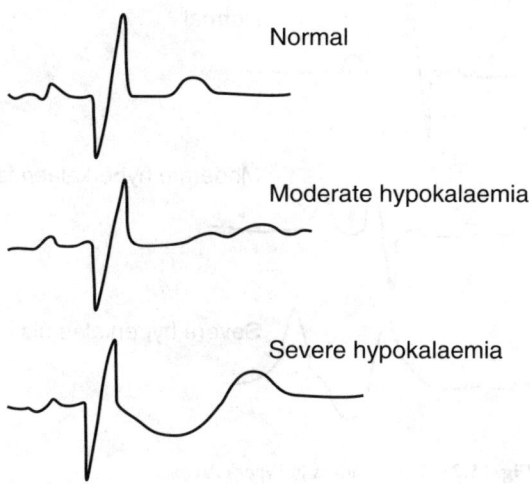

Normal

Moderate hypokalaemia

Severe hypokalaemia

Fig. 15.1 ECG changes in hypokalaemia.

though it has already been emphasized that a normal serum potassium does not by any means exclude significant and perhaps serious potassium depletion.

Treatment of potassium depletion

Obviously, if there is a complex electrolyte distur-bance, the replacement of potassium must be considered in the light of the whole disturbance. This applies particularly to gastrointestinal catastrophes with large loss of gastrointestinal secretions.

In pure potassium deficiency the best treatment for mild or moderate deficiency is to ensure that patients take an adequate amount of potassium in their diet; potassium-rich foods include meat, particularly red meat, fruits and vegetable foods with a high protein content.

In many frail, ill old people, and in those with surgical conditions where feeding by mouth is not feasible, the giving of potassium supplements will be necessary, either orally or parenterally, depending upon clinical circumstances. Intravenous potassium therapy should be reserved for severe potassium depletion with frank hypokalaemia, as is often seen in the following circumstances:

- where life is threatened by the suddenness and severity of potassium loss
- where paralytic ileus has developed
- where frank skeletal muscle paralysis has appeared, especially if the respiratory muscles are involved
- when a patient has clinically important potassium depletion and is unable to take potassium by mouth.

Potassium excess

Potassium excess, which is much rarer than depletion, occurs in people with renal failure. Often there is longstanding low-grade impairment of kidney function, made suddenly worse by an acute infection of renal tissue, treatment with potassium-sparing diuretics (for example, diuretic combinations containing spironolactone or triamterene), or over-enthusiastic supplementation with potassium salts.

As with potassium depletion the brunt of the ill effects falls on cardiac and skeletal muscle, the irritability of which is strongly influenced by the serum potassium concentration.

A considerable rise in serum potassium is often tolerated without symptoms or signs, and up to 7 mmol/l there are usually minimal effects. Beyond this level there are, in parallel with the increasing serum potassium concentration, progressive, abnormal changes in the ECG, in the following sequence:

- high pointed T waves
- reduction of the P wave voltage
- atrial standstill
- widening of the QRS complexes
- lengthening of the QT interval
- development of increasingly serious ventricular arrhythmias
- at serum potassium levels of around 9–11 or more, ventricular fibrillation.

These changes are shown in Figure 15.2.

Treatment of potassium excess

At a serum potassium level of 8 mmol/l, even with minimal ECG change, it is wise to treat the patient, with the aim of preventing more serious abnormalities.

A simple and safe way of reducing serum potassium is to give insulin and glucose; this does not reduce total body potassium but causes a rapid flux of potassium from the extracellular fluid into the cells.

10 units of soluble insulin given subcutaneously, with 50 gm of dextrose infused intravenously as 250 ml of a 20% solution over a period of 1 hour will produce a substantial fall. This procedure can be repeated according to the response, judged by repeated measurements of serum potassium and blood glucose. Care has to be taken to avoid fluid overload with repeated infusion.

If life-threatening ECG changes have already appeared, the risk can be reduced by an intravenous infusion of 10% calcium gluconate given at 2 ml per minute up to a total of 50 ml, together with energetic use of insulin and glucose as described above.

Most patients with advanced renal failure and potassium intoxication will have a metabolic acidosis; this can be temporarily relieved by an intravenous infusion of 1 litre of isotonic sodium bicarbonate, though great care must be taken not to overload the patient with sodium and water.

These measures are all of an emergency nature designed to relieve the immediate risk of death

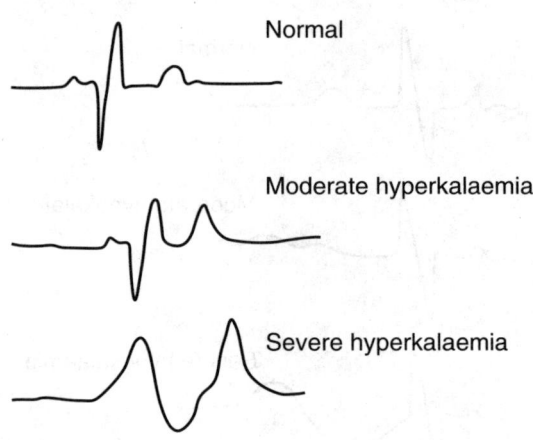

Fig. 15.2   ECG changes in hyperkalaemia.

from cardiac arrhythmia. Once the patient is out of danger from this, the need is to reduce total body potassium. The important measures are:

- Remove any factor which may have precipitated renal failure, such as infection, diuretic drugs or obstructive uropathy.
- Stop potassium supplements if these are being given.
- Give a cation exchange resin orally.
- Plan the longer-term assessment and treatment of the patient's renal failure. This topic is outside the scope of this book but is dealt with in detail in specialist texts.

Diabetes

Introduction

Diabetes mellitus is one of the most important conditions encountered in modern medicine. This is partly because it is so common, partly because of its complexity, and partly because a great deal can be done to help diabetic patients if their condition is managed with care. Diabetes mellitus becomes commoner with age, so it is frequently encountered in geriatric practice. Furthermore, many of the complications of diabetes can cause disability and this brings elderly diabetic patients naturally into the clinical arena of geriatric medicine. Our understanding of the disease is improving, and it is now known that the disease is not simply one of a failure of carbohydrate metabolism, but a more wide-ranging metabolic illness in which hyperglycaemia, though still important for the diagnosis, is only one feature. In this chapter we will concentrate on those aspects of diabetes which are particularly important in geriatric practice.

Classification of diabetes mellitus

The most important distinction is between those patients who are truly lacking in insulin and those in whom there is a resistance to endogenous insulin. The first type have truly insulin-dependent diabetes mellitus (IDDM), and are sometimes also known as Type I or juvenile diabetics. Such patients have the following characteristics:

- The onset of the illness can be at any age, including old age.
- There is a failure to produce insulin in response to carbohydrates.
- Insulin therapy is required

- The onset is often abrupt.
- Patients lapse into diabetic ketoacidosis rapidly if insulin therapy is not given.

The second type, commoner in older people is non-insulin-dependent diabetes mellitus (NIDDM), also known as Type II or maturity onset diabetes. Such patients have the following characteristics:

- The peak instance is between the ages of 55 and 70.
- Patients are often obese.
- The onset is more gradual and ketoacidosis is uncommon.
- The plasma insulin concentration is normal or raised.
- Insulin therapy is usually only required during crises such as severe infections.

The vast majority of elderly diabetics belong to the maturity onset group, but some patients with IDDM survive into old age, and a few develop that condition in old age. The distinction between the two groups is in any case not sharp and maturity-onset diabetes can, during an acute infection or some other general illness, show features more typical of IDDM, particularly ketoacidosis, and then may temporarily require insulin treatment. Middle-aged and elderly patients with NIDDM often present with the clinical triad of diabetes, obesity and hypertension, and have a high prevalence of arteriosclerosis.

This clinical picture is sometimes referred to as the insulin-resistant syndrome and our present understanding of diabetes mellitus of the NIDDM type is that it is a widespread metabolic disease involving not only carbohydrate metabolisms but also the handling of free fatty acids, triglycerides and glycoproteins in which there is also a biochemical disturbance of small vessel basement membrane and endothelium.

Clinical presentation of diabetes in elderly people

Broadly speaking, the mode of presentation in elderly people with diabetes does not differ radically from the presentation in younger patients.

However, listed below are a number of particularly important clinical circumstances in which the previously undiagnosed elderly diabetic patient may present:

- A raised blood sugar or glycosuria is disclosed as an incidental finding during the course of examination for some other disease; the patient is often completely free from diabetic symptoms.
- The diabetes, or in any case the glucose intolerance, is looked for if the patient has one or more of the conditions which can lead to secondary diabetes. Such conditions are outlined in Box 16.1.

Rare in old people is an acute onset in coma and pre-coma. This is only likely to occur in elderly patients when moderately severe but unrecognized diabetes is suddenly transformed into ketoacidosis by a severe infection or generalized illness. The condition develops over some hours or days and is never really abrupt as in hypoglycaemia, another cause of coma in diabetes.

Abdominal pain and vomiting commonly occur and dehydration sets in rapidly, often with rapid, severe loss of visual acuity. When blood sugar levels are very high, the urine will usually contain glucose, and ketones may be detected in urine or on the patient's breath.

Confirmation of the diagnosis

The keystone of laboratory confirmation is measurement of the blood sugar level. The fasting blood sugar of a healthy person usually falls in the range of 3.8–5 mmol/l but values up to 7 mmol/l are considered to be normal in people over the age

---

> ### Box 16.1 Causes of secondary diabetes
>
> - Chronic liver disease.
> - Chronic pancreatitis.
> - Other conditions which destroy the pancreas.
> - Cushing's syndrome.
> - Thyrotoxicosis.
> - Diuretic therapy, particularly thiazides.
> - Corticosteroid therapy.
> - Other rare metabolic conditions such as acromegaly and haemochromatosis.
> - Patients may present with the symptoms of diabetic complications: for example, failing vision from cataracts, intermittent claudication from peripheral vascular disease, peripheral gangrene, angina pectoris, or the symptoms of a neuropathy.
> - Elderly women sometimes present with pruritis vulvae caused by monilial infection.
> - Elderly diabetics sometimes become immobile as a result of diabetic neuropathy or amyotrophy and present with the mobility problem in the first instance.
> - Less common in old people are the classical symptoms of insulin-dependent diabetes; these are polyuria, thirst, a large appetite, weight loss and lethargy.

---

of 70. Ordinary meals cause only a slight rise above the fasting value in health; insulin secretion in response to the meal stows glucose away almost as rapidly as it enters the circulation. For this reason a randomly timed blood sugar which exceeds 8.5 mmol/l is very suggestive of diabetes. When the diagnosis is uncertain, confirmation is best obtained by the standard 75 gm glucose tolerance test (GTT), which deliberately stretches the body's capacity for handling carbohydrate.

It must be emphasized that only a small proportion of patients will require a formal GTT; the vast majority of diabetics can be diagnosed from fasting and random blood sugar estimations.

Protocol for glucose tolerance tests

In the test the patient starves overnight; the following morning a baseline sample is taken, the patient drinks 75 gm of liquid glucose and then the blood sugar is measured at 2 hours, $2\frac{1}{2}$ hours and 3 hours. The upper limits of normal for the GTT in elderly subjects are now generally thought to be somewhat higher than in younger adults. For instance, for elderly subjects the upper limits of glucose in plasma from superficial veins is suggested to be:

- fasting 6.2 mmol/l
- 2 hours 12.2 mmol/l
- $2\frac{1}{2}$ hours 11.1 mmol/l
- 3 hours 10.6 mmol/l.

It is thought that these criteria will detect all but the mildest cases of diabetes whilst avoiding misdiagnosis in healthy old people. Many old people labelled as having mild or borderline diabetes in large community surveys would have been considered nondiabetic by these revised criteria.

Other biochemical measures of diabetes

Though measurement of the blood sugar level and demonstration of abnormally high blood sugar are essential for the diagnosis of diabetes, the longer-term control of blood glucose can be inferred from measuring other blood constituents which are modified by blood glucose levels. Detailed accounts of their chemistry will be found in larger textbooks, though the following two points should be made:

- Blood fructosamine level reflects glycaemic control in the preceding 2–3 weeks.
- Glycosylated haemoglobin level indicates glycaemic control over the preceding few months.

Prevalence of diabetes mellitus in old age

The peak incidence of freshly diagnosed diabetes is in the 55–70 year age band, and as these patients have a life expectancy of about 9 years (approximately 65% of the nondiabetic life expectancy), diabetes is clearly predominantly a disease of elderly people.

The exact prevalence of diabetes in elderly people in the United Kingdom is not known, because large-scale studies based on glucose tolerance tests have not been performed. However, surveys based on random blood sugar measurements and on urine testing for glycosuria suggest that the prevalence is between 4% and 6% of the total of patients above the age of 70, though the incidence of newly diagnosed diabetes continues to rise with age.

The complications of diabetes

Most of the important complications of diabetes are due to the following three mechanisms:

- small vessel disease, microangiopathy
- large vessel disease
- infection.

The speed at which individuals develop such complications varies enormously. Insulin therapy does not protect an individual with certainty from the development of diabetic complications, though there is evidence that strict glycaemic control does modify the rate at which complications progress.

Microangiopathy, affecting mainly capillaries, is a lesion in which there is thickening and loss of structure of the capillary basement membrane. It is not known for certain whether this change is the consequence of impaired carbohydrate metabolism or whether the microangiopathy occurs in parallel with the metabolic disturbance. Though most organs can be affected by the microangiopathy, the three structures which bear the brunt of this complication are as follows:

- the retina
- renal small blood vessels at the level of the glomerulus
- the nerve sheath.

Diabetic retinopathy, nephropathy and neuropathy respectively are the result of such damage. The condition can be seen most clearly by examining the retina, where, in a fully developed example of diabetic retinopathy, there will be microaneurysms, haemorrhages and hard exudates, which can lead to severe loss of vision, particularly if the macula densa is involved. The renal lesion gives rise to progressive renal impairment with a fall in the glomerular filtration rate and a tendency for the glomerulus to leak protein.

Diabetic neuropathy can affect any part of the nervous system and lead to the various complications which are outlined in Figure 16.1.

Diabetes is an important risk factor in the development of atherosclerosis, particularly in patients of European descent. The presence of other risk factors such as hypertension, smoking and hyperlipidaemia accelerate the process. Large vessel disease leads to a very substantial increase in morbidity and mortality, particularly from the following complications:

- stroke
- angina pectoris, myocardial infarction and ischaemic cardiac failure
- lower limb involvement with intermittent claudication and gangrene (a diabetic patient is 50 times more likely to lose a foot from ischaemic gangrene than a nondiabetic patient).

Patients with good glycaemic control probably have no greater tendency to infection than the rest of the population. Those with poorly controlled diabetes do have increased susceptibility to certain infections, and this is probably more of a problem in elderly patients than in the young. The main sites of infection are as follows:

- Urinary tract infection, a particular problem in diabetic women, but seen in both sexes. Lower urinary tract infection, with cystitis, is the most common problem but there is also a higher incidence of pyelonephritis and perinephric abscess.
- Skin infection particularly fungal infection, usually with *Candida albicans*, in moist body clefts, and staphylococcal infection leading to abscesses and carbuncles.
- Infection of mucus membranes with *Candida albicans* particularly in the mouth, pharynx and vagina.
- Respiratory infection, particularly pneumococcal pneumonia. There is also a higher incidence of Gram-negative pneumonia in poorly controlled elderly diabetics, and there is some evidence of an increased tendency to pulmonary tuberculosis.

Some of the most important complications and consequences of diabetes are shown in Box 16.2

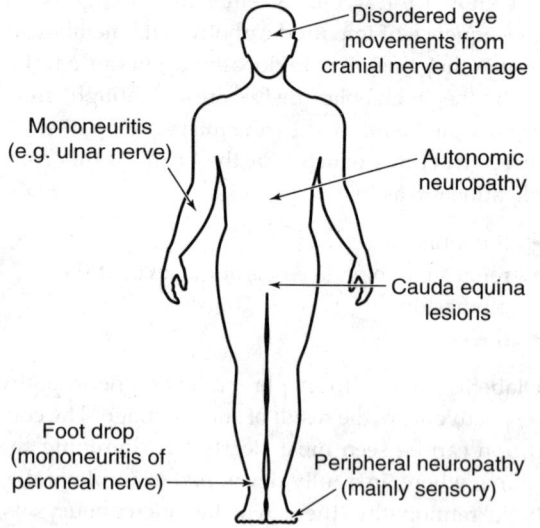

Fig. 16.1 Some important aspects of diabetic neuropathy.

Box 16.2 Complications and consequences of diabetes mellitus

Vascular complications
- Large vessel disease due to obliterative atherosclerosis, particularly of the coronary, cerebral, lower limb and renal vessels
- Microangiopathy at capillary level leading to widespread damage, particularly retinopathy and nephropathy

Eye complications
- Cataract
- Vitreous opacities
- Glaucoma, which is usually secondary to retinopathy
- Diabetic retinopathy with microaneurysms, haemorrhages, hard exudates and new vessel formation

(contd)

Box 16.2 Complications and consequences of diabetes mellitus (contd)

Nervous tissue complications
- Damage to nerves, due to microangiopathy of the vasa nervorum
- Peripheral neuropathy
- Autonomic disturbances, giving rise to postural hypotension, atonic bladder with overflow incontinence, difficulties with swallowing, early morning diarrhoea, impotence, cardiac arrhythmias

Metabolic complications
- Nonketotic hyperosmolar diabetic coma (especially in NIDDM)
- Hyperglycaemic ketoacidotic coma (particularly in IDDM but can be seen in NIDDM)
- Hypoglycaemic coma, usually seen in patients taking insulin or hypoglycaemic drugs

Infection
- Fungal infection, particularly with *Candida albicans* in moist body clefts
- A high attack rate of pneumococcal pneumonia
- A higher incidence of Gram-negative pneumonia
- Staphylococcal infection leading to boils and carbuncles, particularly in patients with very poor diabetic control

Treatment of diabetes

There are four main methods of treating diabetes:

- insulin therapy
- oral hypoglycaemic drugs
- dietary restriction of carbohydrate
- weight reduction in obese people.

The principles are exactly the same for the older patient as for the young. Every patient needs to be considered individually, but broad guidelines can be outlined as follows.

Insulin-dependent diabetes mellitus

By definition insulin therapy is required at all times. The patients are failing to produce endogenous insulin from the pancreatic islet cells. The amount of insulin required will vary from person to person, and in old age a twice-daily regime of insulin usually gives satisfactory control with the minimum of inconvenience. The reader is referred to specialized works on diabetes for more details of insulin therapy.

Non-insulin-dependent diabetes mellitus

Patients who are acutely ill with this condition may need insulin temporarily. Otherwise treatment should consist of weight reduction if the patient is obese, and sensible restriction of carbohydrate in the diet. If such measures do not result in satisfactory control of blood sugar, oral hypoglycaemic agents should be considered. The sulphonylurea agents act partly by stimulating insulin secretion and partly by increasing the number of insulin receptors.

They are very effective but can cause hypoglycaemia if the patient does not eat regularly or if the dose is too high. Short-acting preparations such as tolbutamide and gliclazide are preferable and safer in old people. The biguanide compound metformin probably acts by augmenting muscular glucose uptake and reducing gluconeogenesis. It does not cause hypoglycaemia and is a very useful agent in obese patients. There is a small risk of producing lactic acidosis, particularly in individuals with chronic liver disease. Acarbose can be used as adjunctive therapy or monotherapy alongside dietary restriction.

Acarbose reduces the postprandial glucose peaks by slowing down glucose absorption from the small bowel, as a result of its inhibition of intestinal alpha glucosidase. It does not cause hypoglycaemia when used as monotherapy, but does predispose a patient to hypoglycaemia if used in conjunction with a sulphonylurea agent or insulin.

The treatment of diabetic coma and pre-coma

The acute metabolic disturbance seen in patients with diabetic ketoacidosis or hyperosmolar nonketotic states is a medical emergency.

The treatment is identical in old age as in the young, though great care must be taken with fluid replacement to avoid overloading the circulatory system and precipitating pulmonary oedema. The principles of treatment include correction of salt and water imbalance, insulin therapy, adjustment of the patient's acid-base status and treatment of any underlying precipitating causes such as infection. The student is referred to standard textbooks on emergency medicine and general internal medicine for more detail on the management of acute diabetic states.

Some special aspects of the treatment of diabetes in old age

Insulin therapy. The elderly patient who has had IDDM for many years will probably already be experienced in the use of an insulin syringe, but in those requiring insulin for the first time in later life, detailed instruction followed by checking of their capacity to administer the drug properly is needed.

There is a range of alternative devices, such as insulin pens, on the market which do make things somewhat easier though the need to give proper training and follow-up cannot be overemphasized. Elderly people with cognitive impairment are almost always unable to learn to use any of the insulin injection devices and must have their treatment given by a relative or district nurse, and whenever possible oral drug therapy should be used in such circumstances.

It is also very important to remember that elderly patients, even those who have been highly competent with insulin injection techniques, may become suddenly unable to give their insulin therapy in the event of an acute confusional state, a stroke leading to dyspraxia or weakness, a sudden deterioration in vision or a deterioration in mobility, making it difficult to manage their syringe and drugs.

Hypoglycaemia. Hypoglycaemia is a fairly common and serious complication of diabetes in old people; it occurs not only in patients receiving insulin, but also in those treated with the sulphonylurea hypoglycaemic agents. The risk is particularly high with long-acting drugs such as chlorpropamide and glibenclamide. Lesser degrees of hypoglycaemia would cause a fall-off in competence for self-care, apathy or minor changes in behaviour and mental attitude. More serious degrees lead to stupor or coma which can be fatal if untreated; it is important to remember that the final lapse into unconsciousness often occurs very quickly.

The important features of typical hypoglycaemia are as follows:

- The patient looks unwell with clammy skin and sweating.
- The blood pressure is low.
- There can be puzzling neurological signs, often misinterpreted as strokes these signs can be either bilateral or asymmetrical, and frontal lobe signs with primitive reflexes (such as grasp reflex and extensor planter responses) can be present.
- Estimation of blood sugar will usually indicate a level below 2 mmol/l.

In old age, however, the typical signs of hypoglycaemia can be masked, particularly by the following factors:

- Patients taking betablocker therapy may not get the warning symptoms caused by the surge in adrenalin in response to hypoglycaemia. Therefore, the tremor, tachycardia and feeling of apprehension are absent and the patient is less likely to take action to obtain carbohydrates.
- Older people are likely to lapse into a confusional state at an earlier stage in their hypoglycaemia, and thereby render themselves unable to take appropriate measures to raise their blood sugar.
- There is some evidence to suggest that the intense hunger usually felt by a patient while becoming hypoglycaemic is less or absent in old age, so that the elderly hypoglycaemic patient will be less likely to seek food.

Treatment of hypoglycaemia. Treatment must be given immediately. If the patient is unconscious, an intravenous injection of 50–100 ml of 50% dextrose solution will usually raise the blood sugar sufficiently.

If the diagnosis is correct there will often be an

instantaneous improvement and rapid disappearance of any neurological signs present, though persistence of deep hypoglycaemic coma for 12 hours or more can cause irreversible brain damage.

It is important that if the hypoglycaemia has been produced by a long acting antidiabetic oral drug or long-acting insulin, observation and glucose supplementation will be needed for at least 72 hours, as relapse into coma after successful initial treatment commonly occurs during this period.

Foot care. Many diabetic patients are now managed in specialized diabetic clinics or diabetic centres run in hospital outpatient departments or by their general practitioners. In old people one of the most important aspects of such provision is proper foot care. In elderly diabetic patients the ischaemia, infection and neuropathy which can be a consequence of diabetes can result in extensive damage to the feet.

To minimize foot damage in the elderly diabetic the following precautions should be taken:

- The feet should be inspected at each clinic visit for signs of ulceration, infection, critical ischaemia and advancing neuropathy.
- Patients should be encouraged to inspect their own feet and report immediately to a nurse or medical practitioner if any abnormalities are found.
- The toe nails should be trimmed close and regularly by a chiropodist.
- The feet should be kept scrupulously clean.
- The patient should be encouraged to wear suitable footwear: shoes of soft material are preferred which avoid pinching or putting pressure on the toes.
- Any infection which occurs must be treated vigorously.
- If the foot is ischaemic because of large vessel disease, the patient should be assessed for suitability for bypass grafting.
- There is some evidence to suggest that good control of the blood sugar slows down the rate at which diabetic foot complications occur.

17

Respiratory disease in old age

Introduction

Respiratory disease is responsible for a large proportion of the ill health of elderly people in all societies, and deaths from respiratory causes are also an important feature of old age. For example, in some parts of the United Kingdom, lower respiratory tract infection is the second most common reason for hospital admission after cardiac failure in people over the age of 70. There are, however, some important differences between the mode of presentation and clinical management of a number of common respiratory complaints in old age when compared with younger patients, and these will be outlined in this chapter. Of particular importance is the need to retain a positive approach to the treatment of respiratory conditions in old age; a large percentage of acute respiratory illnesses can be treated successfully even in very frail people so accurate diagnosis of respiratory diseases and thorough management in appropriate cases form an important part of the acute medical management of elderly patients.

Changes in respiratory physiology with age

As age advances a number of structural changes take place in the lung parenchyma and supporting tissues which lead to a progressive change in measurable lung volumes. These are summarized in Figure 17.1. These changes are inevitable, though they are accelerated by other factors such as industrial pollution and smoking. As a consequence, the amount of lung tissue available to take part in the respiratory process falls and this is one of the fac-

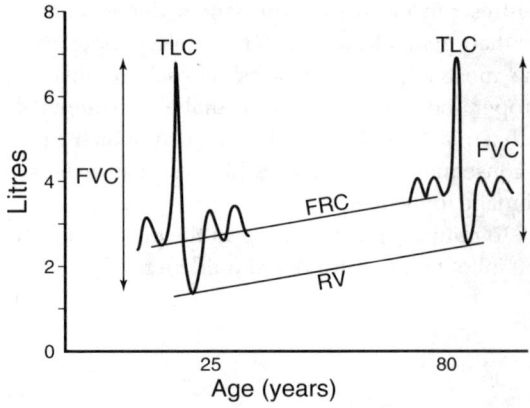

Fig. 17.1 Changes in lung volumes with age. FVC = forced vital capacity; TLC = total lung capacity; FRC = functional residual capacity; RV = residual volume (from Brocklehurst J C, Tallis R C, Fillit H M (eds) Textbook of geriatric medicine and gerontology. Churchill Livingstone, Edinburgh).

tors which impose a limit on respiratory performance in old age. There is also evidence that the ventilatory and respiratory centre responses to hypoxia, carbon dioxide and respiratory loading (obstruction or restriction) are also reduced with age, though these factors are not thought to cause major changes to the normal physiological response in a normal elderly person. Perhaps one of the most important ways of visualizing the fall in respiratory reserves with age is to consider the ability of the individual to assimilate oxygen under exercise conditions. In a number of extensive cross-sectional and longitudinal studies it has been found that in healthy individuals the maximum achievable oxygen consumption ($\dot{V}O_2$ max) begins to fall quite rapidly after the age of 60 as a result of changes in the respiratory and cardiac symptoms with age.

Contributing to this fall in $\dot{V}O_2$ max are the following factors:

- reduction in respirable lung volumes which limits ventilatory capacity
- an increasing mismatch of ventilation to perfusion in the lung parenchyma
- limits on cardiac output imposed by a progressive fall in the maximum achievable heart rate and stroke volume.

It can be seen in Figures 13.2 and 13.3 (see pp.106 and 107) that the fall in $\dot{V}O_2$ max imposes a ceiling on cardiorespiratory performance with advancing age. This decline will occur even in individuals who keep themselves in good cardiorespiratory condition by taking exercise, though there is ample evidence that taking such exercise enables individuals to retain their best possible $\dot{V}O_2$ max. It can be seen clearly that superimposed illnesses are more likely to cause respiratory failure in old age compared within the young because the failure threshold of the respiratory system will be passed at an earlier stage. This is one of the reasons why prompt action is required in the management of acute cardiorespiratory illnesses in elderly patients, even when the superimposed illness appears superficially to be relatively mild.

Pneumonia

While there is no evidence that elderly people are particularly prone to upper respiratory tract infection, there is no doubt that the incidence of serious lower respiratory tract infections increases steeply with age and frailty. Consequently, pneumonia is one of the commonest reasons for admission of an elderly person to hospital, one of the commonest complications of other debilitating medical conditions and a common cause of death. The clinical presentation may be identical to that which is typical of younger patients, with a fairly abrupt onset of fever with rigors, cough, the production of sputum, which is sometimes blood-stained, and breathlessness. On the other hand, as people become older and frailer, and particularly when there is other coexistent pathology, the clinical pre-

sentation of pneumonia can be very different. Some of the most important features of pneumonia in old age include:

- A large number of patients present with an acute confusional state.
- Typical respiratory symptoms may be absent or difficult to elicit.
- Cardiac failure is a common complication and the patients may present with the symptoms and signs of cardiac failure dominating the clinical scene.
- Other geriatric giant presentations are not uncommon, including falls, sudden reduction in mobility, incontinence and general failure to cope.

Similarly, the physical signs can be classical, and an elderly person with lobar consolidation might have the usual physical signs of dullness to percussion, bronchial breathing and increased vocal resonance over the affected part. However, this is the exception in pneumonia in elderly people. More commonly, the physical signs are much less clear-cut. Nevertheless, the following physical signs can be very helpful:

- Though some elderly people with pneumonia are genuinely afebrile, research has shown that at least 80% will have some rise in body temperature, providing temperature is recorded properly.
- A respiratory rate elevated above 24 p.m. is abnormal and though not specific for pneumonia should prompt a search for that diagnosis.
- Auscultation often reveals reduction of air entry and coarse crackles over an affected lung base. Because basal lung crackles are so common in elderly people, the finding of asymmetry of this physical sign is quite useful.
- If a specimen of sputum can be examined it is often yellow or green in patients with bacterial infection in the respiratory tract.

In an elderly person suspected of having pneumonia, the most important investigation is a chest radiograph, and although classical lobar consolidation is relatively uncommon, there is often evidence of patchy consolidation in the affected lobe. The radiograph also enables the clinician to look for radiological evidence of cardiac failure. The majority of patients mount a neutrophil leucocytosis, though this can be relatively undramatic. It is useful to get an estimation of the urea and electrolyte level, partly to assess dehydration and partly to find out whether the patient is becoming hyponatraemic as a result of inappropriate antidiuretic hormone (ADH) secretion. Sputum culture is relatively unhelpful, unless a very good specimen can be obtained, though blood cultures can prove useful, particularly in the diagnosis of pneumococcal pneumonia.

The type of infecting organism will vary according to prevailing epidemic conditions, the patient's general clinical state, and whether the patient was admitted from home or an institution or acquired the pneumonia in hospital. In general the following points should be made:

- The commonest cause of pneumonia in elderly people is *Streptococcus pneumoniae*.
- Patients debilitated by neurological disease, such as stroke or motor neuron disease, have a relatively high incidence of pneumonia caused by Gram-negative organisms and anaerobes.
- Debilitated patients who acquire their pneumonia in hospital have a high incidence of Gram-negative anaerobic pneumonia.
- Atypical pneumonia due to organisms such as *Chlamydia pneumoniae* and mycoplasma pneumoniae is probably no more common in old people than in young adults.
- Some elderly people with tuberculosis present with an apparently acute pneumonia, or with a superimposed pyogenic pneumonia.

Management and treatment

The general management includes the following:

- Oxygen supplementation should be given to hypoxic patients.
- There should be adequate fluid replacement, though care must be taken not to give excessive fluids and precipitate heart failure.
- There should be optimal control of coexistent pathologies, particularly cardiac failure, diabetes mellitus and reversible air flow obstruction.

- In relatively immobile patients, precautions should be taken to avoid pressure sores, and subcutaneous heparin may be needed as prophylaxis against deep venous thrombosis and pulmonary embolism.
- Patients who are acutely confused with aggression and high levels of anxiety run the risk of exhausting themselves and sometimes require tranquillizer therapy; thioridazine and haloperidol are useful in this context, though care must be taken not to oversedate the patient and suppress respiratory drive.

In very ill elderly patients a decision needs to be made whether to give intensive therapy support, and this will depend very much on the overall clinical context. For example, it would not be appropriate to treat pneumonia with vigour in a patient dying from widespread malignancy. In otherwise healthy elderly people with severe pneumonia very good results can be obtained with intensive therapy support. The most important indications for referral to intensive care are persistent hypotension despite fluid replacement and oxygen, and persistent hypoxia; a short period of continuous positive airways pressure or assisted ventilation can make a tremendous difference to an old person becoming exhausted with severe pneumonia.

Antibiotic therapy. The choice of antibiotic therapy will depend upon prevailing bacteriological patterns and the availability of various drugs. In the United Kingdom the British Thoracic Society guidelines indicate that mild community-acquired lower respiratory tract infection can be treated in the first place with ampicillin or amoxycillin, and moderate or severe community-acquired pneumonia should be treated with a second-generation cephalosporin plus erythromycin.

Beyond this it is very much a case of using clinical judgement, reinforced by whatever bacteriological evidence can be obtained. Generally speaking, if staphylococcal infection is suspected, an anti-staphylococcal drug such as flucloxacillin should be added; if Gram-negative pneumonia is suspected, a third-generation cephalosporin or aminoglycoside antibiotic will be needed; and if anaerobic organisms might be present it is usual to add metronidazole to the drug regimen. It is sensible to involve a microbiologist in difficult antibiotic decisions whenever possible.

Asthma

Asthma is an important illness in old age. Most people with asthma in this age group have been asthmatic for most of their life, though a few people develop the symptoms and signs of asthma for the first time in old age. The typical symptoms of breathlessness, wheezing and cough are the commonest complaints of an asthmatic elderly person, though as with most other severe medical conditions, acute, moderate or severe asthma can present in an atypical way. The diagnosis of asthma should always be considered as a possibility in older people who present with:

- wheezy dyspnoea, particularly when there is no history of cigarette smoking or of chronic airflow limitation
- limited exercise tolerance associated with cough and chest tightness
- presentation with acute confusion, immobility, incontinence or other geriatric problems, particularly when the patient has unexplained hypoxia, and expiratory rhonchi are heard on examination of the chest.

The diagnosis is confirmed, as in younger people, by demonstrating reversibility of airflow obstruction when a beta 2 agonist, such as salbutamol, is administered by aerosol. A 15% improvement in the forced expiratory volume in 1 second is virtually diagnostic, and a 10% improvement is highly suggestive of asthma. Some patients will only respond when given a trial of corticosteroid therapy.

Treatment of an acute attack of asthma in an elderly person is conducted in the same way as for a young adult, as follows:

- Admission to hospital is required for all but the mild cases.
- Monitoring of oxygen saturation, with oxygen supplementation, is essential.
- Bronchodilator drugs are administered by nebulizer and face mask.
- Patients with moderate or severe asthma will require corticosteroid therapy to suppress bronchial inflammation as quickly as possible.

- Elderly patients with acute severe asthma become fatigued very early in the illness, so referral to an intensive care unit for ventilatory support should occur even earlier in an elderly patient than in a young one.
- Coexistent pathology must be treated to optimize the patient's general medical condition.
- All patients should have a chest radiograph shortly after admission to hospital to rule out a pneumothorax.
- The majority of elderly patients with acute severe asthma respond very well to such a regimen, and can then be established on long-term maintenance therapy. This should also follow the usual guidelines, though very few elderly asthmatics benefit from treatment with chromoglycate.

The mainstay of maintenance therapy is as follows:

- Regular inhaled corticosteroid should be given, using the lowest dose possible to keep the patient in remission.
- Inhaled beta 2 agonist therapy should be given when required to relieve transient symptoms.
- Elderly patients sometimes find it difficult to detect a deterioration in the state of their asthma, and in such cases inhaled bronchodilator therapy should be given regularly, usually as a combination of a beta 2 agonist such as salbutamol with an anticholinergic agent: for example, ipatropium bromide. Very few patients require oral corticosteroid maintenance therapy. Some patients obtain additional symptomatic benefit at night by taking aminophylline tablets when they go to bed, though care must be taken not to cause aminophylline toxicity. Elderly asthmatics should stop smoking and if their attacks of asthma are precipitated by any obvious allergens, which is unusual, these should be avoided.

While most normal elderly patients can learn to use a standard metered dose inhaler without much difficulty, particularly if it is attached to a large volume spacer device, some patients find this very difficult, and special provision will have to be made for patients who fall into the following groups:

- Patients with definite cognitive impairment are unable to use a standard metered dose inhaler, though those with mild dementia can sometimes learn consistently to use simpler inhaler devices.
- Patients who are dyspraxic as a result of cerebrovascular disease, particularly stroke, are usually unable to use an inhaler.
- Patients with weak or painful hands are unable to trigger an ordinary inhaler and will require an alternative device.
- Patients who have very poor vision will require special training.

A range of special devices is available to help people with these problems obtain inhaled respiratory therapy, and there is no need for them to be listed in detail here. The most important point is that an appropriate device needs to be selected for the individual patient, thorough training in the use of the device by a nurse or doctor is required, and patients must be followed up to make sure that they have retained the information and are still using the inhaler properly. Failure to use inhaler therapy properly is an important cause of relapse of asthma in old age, the other important factor being respiratory infection.

Chronic airflow limitation

Chronic airflow limitation is a very common condition in elderly patients, particularly men, with a high prevalence in industrialized parts of the world, where the main aetiological factor is cigarette smoking, though industrial and other atmospheric pollution may contribute. The underlying pathological process is emphysema, and there is often chronic inflammatory damage to the airways themselves.

Typically, both the FEV_1 (volume expired in 1 second) and FVC (forced vital capacity) are reduced, the former more than the latter, giving the typical obstructive pattern on respiratory function tests. Mild chronic airflow limitation causes few problems in elderly people, though there is a higher proneness to develop pneumonia. On the other hand, moderate and severe chronic airflow limitation can cause significant reduction in exercise tolerance and is a major predisposing factor for pneumonia, particularly in the winter.

The main symptoms are breathlessness and wheezing, and there is usually, though not invariably, the production of clear or grey sputum on most days. When superimposed infection in the airways or lung parenchyma is present, the patient becomes iller, and in old age may present with predominantly geriatric problems rather than respiratory. During infective exacerbations the sputum is often yellow or green, the respiratory rate is usually raised, physical signs in the chest are very unreliable in this context, though asymmetrical crackles suggest basal pneumonia, and a chest radiograph is often useful to help clarify the clinical state.

The management of acute infective exacerbations of chronic airflow limitation are dealt with in detail in major textbooks, though the main elements of treatment are summarized in Box 17.1.

Box 17.1 Treatment of acute exacerbation of chronic airflow limitation

- Antibiotic therapy is necessary if bacterial infection is suspected or proven.
- Administration of bronchodilator drugs by nebulizer is often helpful; there is usually some subjective improvement in symptoms, even when measurable reversibility is not detected on pulmonary function testing.
- Oxygen supplementation is often required, though care must be taken not to cause carbon dioxide retention in chronically hypoxic patients with a low respiratory drive. It is usual to administer 24% oxygen in the first place.
- Patients should remain as mobile as possible, and very immobile patients may require prophylaxis against deep venous thrombosis with subcutaneous heparin and lower limb compression stockings.
- Some patients might require assisted ventilation, though it can be very difficult to remove people from mechanical ventilators if their preceding chronic airflow limitation was severe.
- Coexisting pathology, particularly cardiac failure, requires careful monitoring and optimal treatment.

The longer-term management centres around trying to reduce the rate of decline of airways function, obtaining the maximum symptomatic benefit from bronchodilator therapy, and remaining as physically active as possible. Important measures to these ends are listed in Box 17.2.

The same proviso about long-term maintenance

Box 17.2 Long-term management of chronic airflow limitation

- Patients should be advised to stop smoking; even late in the disease process this can be beneficial.
- Administration of a bronchodilator drug has been shown to give symptomatic benefit in some patients, even when no reversibility is demonstrated on pulmonary function testing.
- Some patients obtain symptomatic benefit from taking aminophylline derivatives.
- Patients should be encouraged to take as much exercise as possible within the context of their respiratory dysfunction and as other physical problems allow.
- Patients should be advised to seek medical help immediately if they develop any signs or symptoms of superimposed chest infection.

---

inhaler therapy, mentioned above for asthmatic patients, also applies in patients with chronic airflow limitation. The final point to be made is that great care must be taken not to diagnose mistakenly chronic airflow limitation in patients who really have asthma. If there is any doubt about the diagnosis, a trial of steroid therapy and reversibility testing must be carried out.

Tuberculosis

The incidence of tuberculosis varies enormously in different parts of the world. In northern Europe and North America there is evidence that the incidence may be rising in frail elderly people, probably due to reactivation of dormant tuberculosis as cell-mediated immunity declines. It is also an important condition in elderly immigrants from parts of the world where the prevalence is very high, for example, South Asia, and parts of Southeast Asia and Africa. Pulmonary tuberculosis is the usual form in elderly indigenous Europeans, though nonpulmonary tuberculosis is relatively common in the immigrant Asian population.

The treatment of tuberculosis in elderly people is along the same lines as in a younger age group and the reader is referred to specialist textbooks for details.

Sensory problems: blindness and deafness

Blindness

Failing vision comes second in Shakespeare's list of the penalties of old age: 'sans teeth, sans eyes, sans taste, sans everything'. Indeed, in the United Kingdom and similar countries about 75% of people who are registered as blind or as having significantly impaired vision are over the age of 65.

Total or near-total blindness in old people is always due to structural disease, either of the eye itself or of the nervous pathways concerned with vision, but a mild degree of visual impairment is an intrinsic effect of ageing, and so by definition is inevitable if the old person lives long enough.

Age-determined changes in vision

These changes consist of:

- presbyopia – reduced power of accommodation
- reduction of visual acuity
- impaired dark adaptation.

Accommodation is the ability to form a sharp image of an object on the retina, over a range of distances from the eye, and is achieved by increasing the convexity of the lens. The extent to which this can be done falls progressively throughout adult life and is closely correlated with age: at 20 years the lens has an accommodative range of about 10 dioptres. (A dioptre is the optical strength of a lens with a focal length of 1 metre.) This value falls to less than 2 dioptres at age 60 on average and is as low as 0.75 in people above the age of 70. Symptoms of accommodative stress particularly

discomfort on attempting near vision, begin at age 40–50. There are two main reasons for this effect:

- The equatorial diameter of the lens increases more than its thickness, so the radius of curvature becomes larger.
- The lens substance becomes less elastic with age, which reduces the amount by which the focal length of the lens can be changed.

These changes cause longsightedness in old people, which is the condition known as presbyopia. Visual acuity is the equivalent of resolving power in a piece of optical equipment. It attains its best value at 20, then remains more or less constant till age 50, after which it gradually deteriorates until the age of around 70, and then a much more rapid decline occurs so that people over the age of 80 have about one-quarter of the visual acuity of people at the age of 20. Nevertheless, at age 70 about one-third of old people will still have virtually full vision, once suitable correction for refraction has been made, and at the age of 80 the figure is still about 10%. The changes responsible for this are not fully understood. Senile myosis is one factor; the pupil area is substantially smaller in old people, so the amount of light admitted to the eye at a given illumination is reduced, while the depth of focus is increased, exactly as in the stop of a camera. Light scattering and absorption in the lens and vitreous body also contribute, but these two effects are not the whole explanation; it is very likely that central processing of visual information is also impaired, possibly even at the level of the visual cortex.

While these intrinsic age changes cause some loss of vision, the remaining faculty is often perfectly adequate for the old person's needs, especially if illumination is at the optimal level.

Blindness acquired in old age

The commonest pathological causes of blindness acquired in later life are:

- cataracts
- glaucoma
- senile macular degeneration
- diabetic retinopathy
- optic tract lesions complicating stroke
- important but less common conditions include cranial arteritis, hypertensive retinopathy and visual cortex infarction.

Clinical examination

While detailed examination of visual function and eye disease is obviously a specialist matter, simple clinical methods give much information and should include the following:

- examination of the external eye, for detection of corneal opacities, iritis, pupil changes and signs of previous operations
- crude tests of visual acuity: the ability to read print of various sizes on a card
- ophthalmoscopic examination, for detection of lens opacities as well as changes in the retina including the blood vessels, macula densa and optic disc
- assessment of visual fields by confrontation.

Cataract

Cataract does not usually cause total blindness, but gives rise to a mild or moderate visual loss of slow onset. Cataracts are due to local irregularities in the lens structure, either in its nucleus or cortex, which are opaque to light.

They can be detected by focusing the ophthalmoscope on the lens rather than the retina, and appear as greyish-black dots or lines, spidery figures or 'cuneiform' opacities. Accurate assessment

requires examination with the narrow beam of a slit lamp. As already mentioned, the lens continues to lay down new fibres throughout life; the most recent are on the outside, like the layers of an onion, and optical discontinuities or 'disjunction stripes' accumulate throughout life, much like the growth rings of a tree.

In some individuals cataract is probably a genetically determined exaggeration of this process. However, since these alterations in lens morphology occur in all individuals, the formation of cataracts becomes extremely common in the very old. Some conditions render the patient particularly liable to develop cataracts. These include:

- diabetes mellitus
- hyperuricaemia
- corticosteroid treatment
- chronic renal failure.

Cataract is often bilateral, though there is frequently a considerable difference between the two sides. The disease does not cause total blindness, but can cause severe loss of vision.

The management of cataract is a matter for the ophthalmologist. Patients with nuclear cataract often show increasing myopia and a change of glasses is often adequate treatment. Dilatation of the pupil, provided there is no risk of glaucoma, may also succeed.

In countries where the necessary services and technology are generally available, operative treatment consists of removal of the affected lens and implantation of a lens prosthesis. When artificial lenses are not available the refraction defect caused by removing the natural lens can be compensated by glasses, usually with an optical strength of about + 10 dioptres plus correction for astigmatism. These corrections may cause spherical distortion and magnification of the image, which is not usually a problem when a lens prosthetic implant is used.

There are some surgical risks attached to cataract operation including retinal detachment and glaucoma in the operated eye, which make ophthalmic surgeons conservative in their approach to cataract in some old people, especially if the other eye has adequate corrected vision.

Glaucoma

This condition is characterized by a rise in intra-ocular pressure. The normal pressure is between 14 and 20 mmHg. If intra-ocular pressure is prolonged it can cause compression of the optic nerve head with consequent impairment of visual fields and visual acuity.

Two types of glaucoma are recognized, as described below.

Closed-angle glaucoma

In this condition the aqueous humour of the anterior chamber of the eye cannot drain away properly because the iris is jammed up against the filtration angle.

Consequently, Schlemm's canal is closed and the normal function of the trabecular mesh is impeded. The intra-ocular pressure rises to 45 mmHg or more. This type of glaucoma is predisposed to by a shallow anterior chamber, usually because of a large lens, and a naturally acute filtration angle.

There are various patterns of clinical presentation, as follows.

Acute glaucoma. There is severe pain in the eye, sometimes with vomiting, blurred vision and a cloudy oedematous cornea. The pupil is dilated, oval and nonreactive to light.

Subacute glaucoma. There are often repeated minor prodromal attacks, in which there is pain in the eye. This is usually less severe than in acute glaucoma. There is often blurring of vision and rainbow haloes on looking at lights.

Chronic closed-angle glaucoma. This presents without ocular pain, haloes or blurring of vision, but there is a gradual loss of vision due to optic nerve compression. This type of glaucoma may well be precipitated by careless dilatation of a pupil.

Treatment

Treatment of the acute attack is an emergency which should be dealt with in an ophthalmology ward and consists of intensive attempts to constrict the pupils with drugs such as pilocarpine. If this fails, the carbonic anhydrase inhibitor acetazo-lamide can be given intramuscularly, and if this in turn is unsuccessful, an operation may be required.

Chronic closed-angle glaucoma will need operative management with an iridectomy or one of the more recently developed drainage operations.

Open-angle glaucoma

This condition is due to impaired reabsorption of the aqueous humour and is of unknown cause. The patient usually presents because of visual impairment, or the condition is discovered at routine examination through the detection of a 'cupped' optic disc by an optician, ophthalmologist or general clinician. Treatment is again a specialist matter; if the patient has no material visual loss, medical measures for control of the intra-ocular pressure will be tried first. On the other hand, if the visual field loss is extensive and enlarging, a drainage operation will be required.

Senile macular degeneration

Since the macula densa is concerned with central vision, its 'degeneration', seen as whitish or grey mottling in the macular and perimacular regions, often with some pigmentation, causes serious visual loss; the onset, fortunately, is fairly slow.

The condition is probably hereditary in most cases. The only treatment possible is strong reading glasses and a magnifying glass for close work. Patients can often walk reasonably safely but are at a loss with work requiring detailed vision.

Diabetic retinopathy

As with younger patients, diabetic retinopathy can be very severe in the presence of quite mild diabetes. It is revealed by the characteristic microaneurysms, haemorrhages, hard exudates and new vessel formation. Loss of vision ensues rapidly when the macula densa is heavily affected. Good glycaemic control is thought to be helpful, though there is enormous variation between individual patients. Laser photocoagulation of areas of neovascularization is very helpful in controlling the rate of progress of diabetic retinopathy.

Visual field defects

A common visual problem in old people is an homonymous hemianopia or quadrantanopia complicating a cerebrovascular accident. In the typical case, the field of vision is lost to the midline in each eye, on the same side as the limb weakness. Providing the old person is capable of cooperating, the lesion can be detected by the simple confrontation test.

Cranial arteritis

This is one of the few causes of acutely developing total blindness in old people and is to some extent preventable. The importance of early recognition and treatment with corticosteroids has been stressed in the chapter on the nervous system.

The effects of blindness on old people

A person who becomes blind in early life, and grows old with the disability, will already have life confidently organized, but blindness occurring out of the blue in an old person is a catastrophe which very often obliterates self-confidence and makes for total dependence on others.

If there is a caring relative with whom the old person can live, much can be done in the way of social rehabilitation, but for those living alone, complete self-care is rarely possible. Therefore, a great deal of thought needs to be put into the arrangement to support blind elderly people and their relatives if an attempt is to be made by the patient to live as independently as possible.

Learning to read Braille is beyond the capacity of most elderly blind people, though the large letter 'Moon' system can be mastered by some. In many countries, audiotape talking books are available, and in the United Kingdom, an old person who is registered blind can apply through social services departments to the British Talking Book Services for the blind. Similar services are available in a number of other countries.

Hearing and deafness

One of the most obvious attributes of ageing is an increasing difficulty in hearing. To what extent this is an age change and to what extent it is due to age-associated disease varies from patient to patient. The possible causes of impairment of hearing with age are many. Some examples would include:

- the primary degeneration of the organ of Corti with loss of epithelial nerve cells commencing in middle life
- changes in the sensory cells of the cochlea
- degenerative changes in the afferent and efferent nerve fibres
- degeneration in the spiral ganglion cells in the base of the cochlea
- loss of elasticity in the basilar membrane of the cochlea and in the tympanic membrane.

In addition to these effects on the organ of hearing itself, there can be abnormalities in other structures involved in hearing, such as:

- the blood supply to the neurosensory receptor mechanism
- degenerative change or vascular damage to the auditory pathways and temporal lobe of the brain.

It seems clear, therefore, that age change and hearing may well be multifactoral in cause. Not only have several age-related and pathological changes been identified as causes but there are also several types of hearing loss occurring with advancing age. These are discussed opposite.

Presbyacusis

This is a loss of pure tone hearing in the higher frequencies. It is an age-related phenomenon.

Abnormal loudness perception

This is usually seen in people with presbyacusis. Approximately 60% of patients with presbyacusis will experience hypersensitivity to very loud speech, such that an intensity level which will be acceptable to the normal person becomes unacceptable to the patient with presbyacusis.

Tinnitus

This has been shown to increase in prevalence from about 3% in the second decade of life to over 10% in the sixth decade, though tinnitus is not necessarily associated with hearing loss.

Impairment of sound localization

This may affect hearing by impairing the ability of the person to discriminate among the sounds heard in a noisy environment. Simply identifying the loss of high-frequency tones by audiometry carried out in a soundproof room will not, therefore, necessarily give a good assessment of the hearing difficulties experienced by old people.

In addition, some tests involving the selection of one out of a number of sound signals will be required. Lip reading may also form a compensatory mechanism for some hearing loss.

Different surveys have indicated different levels of hearing difficulties among the aged population. In people over the age of 70, the figure seems to lie somewhere between 12% and 30%, depending partly on the criteria used, though there is no doubt that a sizeable proportion of the elderly population have significant hearing loss. For this reason, assessment of the cause of hearing impairment is worth while in all elderly patients. A few important general steps in this assessment are as follows:

- First exclude wax in the outer ear. Some studies have shown that about one-third of elderly patients who complain of reduced hearing have excessive wax in the external auditory meatus and in a proportion of those patients its removal is all that is required to restore an acceptable level of hearing.
- The second step is to provide an adequate electronic hearing aid and careful instruction in its use, together with follow-up support and encouragement.

Hearing aids have many limitations, since increasing the volume of speech will not necessarily increase its intelligibility, and abnormal loudness perception may limit the degree of amplification which is acceptable. A checklist for patients with hearing aids is given in Box 18.1.

The use of two hearing aids, one in each ear, is better than one and best results will be obtained in face-to-face conversation. The effect of a hearing aid in listening to what is being said at a distance is to pick up all the other extraneous sounds in the room. The result is akin to that of a tape recorder which has been placed to pick up group conversation and which seems particularly to magnify extraneous sounds such as doors banging and people coughing.

It is important to find out just how much a person is being handicapped by their loss of hearing. For example, a person may have found it very difficult to take advantage of radio and television, in which case it is possible to provide special adaptors which can provide a direct input from the televi-

---

Box 18.1 Checklist for advising patients with hearing aids

- Make sure the earpiece is not blocked with wax.
- Make sure the battery is live.
- Check the hearing aid is switched on and properly adjusted.
- Make sure there are no electrical disconnections.
- Check that your patient can fit the earpiece correctly.
- Encourage your patient to use the hearing aid as much as possible to get accustomed to it.

sion or radio to an earpiece or the patient's own hearing aid. Similarly, if a patient is unable to hear a door bell, it is useful to substitute this with a flashing light. Drugs have nothing to offer in the management of presbyacusis.

Ménière's disease

This is a common condition in old age and is the result of degenerative changes in the cochlear aque-duct leading to endolymphatic hydrops. In its acute form it presents with vertigo and tinnitus, and in the more chronic case the vertigo tends to settle down and the patient has persistent tinnitus with loss of hearing on that side. It is sometimes bilateral, in which case the hearing loss can be substantial. Patients who are troubled with vertigo are often helped by betahistine, though this will not modify the hearing loss.

19

Nutrition

Introduction

The impairment of nutrition in elderly people may present as undernutrition – that is an insufficient intake of essential nutrients, or as overnutrition – that is, obesity. Disorders of nutrition in either of these conditions may lead to disease. On the other hand, they may be the result of disease. The most important patterns of nutritional impairment seen in elderly patients in Europe and North America are:

- protein and calorie undernutrition leading to weight loss and wasting
- inadequate intake of specific dietary factors such as vitamin D or iron
- excessive calorie intake with weight gain leading to obesity.

In elderly people it is important to consider, first of all, whether there is any evidence that nutrition is impaired, secondly, what are the associated factors with individual nutrients; and thirdly, how nutrition may be improved or maintained in old people.

The nutritional state can be assessed by three general methods:

- by measuring, usually estimating, dietary intake
- by measuring blood or tissue levels of various nutrients
- by looking for clinical evidence of undernutrition or overnutrition.

Only the last of these is likely to give firm evidence of undernutrition since both the dietary intake and blood and tissue levels may vary with age and as a result of associated diseases. Indeed, authorities vary in their definitions of malnutrition, though one which is of practical use states that malnutrition is 'a disturbance of normal function due to lack or excess of one or more nutrients'.

Diet and longevity

Before considering the clinical aspects of malnutrition it is worth mentioning some of the observations in relation to ageing and dietary intake.

Well-known experiments with rats, comparing one group maintained on a restricted diet throughout their lives with another allowed to eat ad lib, showed that those on the restricted diet had a longer lifespan, although they looked thin and less attractive.

If the overfeeding was restricted to the period of growth, it hastened maturity but shortened life. If, on the other hand, the animals were fed a restricted diet until maturity and thereafter were allowed to overfeed, the incidence of disease in old age seemed to be increased. Of course, it is not known whether a direct extrapolation from these experiments can be used to give us a better understanding of human nutrition in relation to ageing, though it is well established that people with the more severe forms of overnutrition with obesity have a higher incidence of certain pathological states which can potentially shorten life: for example, diabetes mellitus, hypertension and vascular disease.

Dietary surveys in old age

Such surveys would throw up very different results in different parts of the world. Some of the most thorough surveys have been performed in Britain and North America so it is important to interpret the results of dietary surveys in old age within the social and cultural context prevailing. There must also be care in interpreting the results of questionnaire and diary surveys of diet, as there is ample evidence that the accuracy of surveys based on this type of information-gathering is not always reliable.

Nevertheless, in a large survey in the United Kingdom, the most striking result was that less than 3% of the general elderly population living at home were regarded as malnourished. In the majority, the intake of energy, protein, calcium, iron and essential vitamins was considered to be satisfactory. On the other hand, surveys of ill elderly people have shown that certain vulnerable groups run the risk of being severely undernourished and can therefore be identified as particularly at risk of malnutrition.

The dietary intake in healthy old people only diminishes slightly with advancing age, though it tends to fall very considerably in those suffering from disabling diseases. The groups of patients known to be particularly at risk of undernutrition are listed in Box 19.1.

If we consider the individual nutrients, protein nutrition seems to be little affected by age unless the patient is very ill or debilitated. In affluent countries this probably reflects the general availability and relatively low cost of protein-containing foods. Some insight has been gained into problems with vitamin nutrition in elderly patients, which can be summarized as follows:

- *The 'B' group vitamins (thiamine, pyridoxine and nicotinic acid)*. These show diminished blood levels in disabled old people which can be restored to normal by adequate supplementation. In the main, these low blood levels of B vitamins are not matched by clinical signs of subnutrition, but in a number of cases, angular stomatitis, cheilosis (red, denuded, scaly epithelium in the line of closure of the lips) and a sodden appearance of the dorsum of the tongue are associated with these deficiencies and can be reversed by supplementation. Angular stomatitis and tongue changes in particular are both

---

Box 19.1 Those at risk of undernutrition

- People with debilitating physical illnesses such as severe rheumatoid arthritis, severe chronic cardiac failure and malignant disease with anorexia
- Patients in hospital with acute severe medical illnesses such as pneumonia, septicaemia and acute heart failure
- Patients with neurological lesions which prevent or inhibit swallowing, such as stroke with dysphagia, conditions impairing consciousness, severe Parkinson's disease and motor neuron disease
- Patients with severe psychiatric conditions, particularly depression and uncontrolled psychoses
- People with advanced dementia, or those with milder dementia if still living alone
- Frail elderly men living alone, who are more likely to be undernourished than elderly women living alone.

---

multifactoral and may be caused by fungal infestation in the mouth and indeed by wearing ill-fitting dentures.

- *Vitamin C, ascorbic acid*. Blood levels of this vitamin again tend to be low in the disabled elderly, particularly those in hospital, but it is uncommon to find evidence of frank scurvy. Scurvy has occasionally been seen in the United Kingdom in frail, elderly men living alone who are taking a very restricted diet, virtually devoid of fruit and vegetables.
- *Vitamin B_{12} and folic acid*. Vitamin B_{12} deficiency due to inadequate dietary intake is extremely rare and is only likely to be seen in people with very unusual diets. Most people with vitamin B_{12} deficiency have atrophic gastritis or disease in the terminal ileum. On the other hand, dietary folic acid deficiency is relatively common, particularly in frail elderly patients whose diet contains little vegetable matter, and is also a fairly common finding in elderly people who abuse alcohol.

- *Vitamin A*. There is no evidence of vitamin A deficiency among old people in the United Kingdom, the rest of Europe and North America.
- *Vitamin D*. Adequate vitamin D status requires both sufficient intake and also exposure to sunlight, and this latter factor may be very important among elderly people in Great Britain, particularly during the winter months. Lack of vitamin D leads to osteomalacia and there is some evidence that osteomalacia in Britain is more common in the months of January to June than July to December.

The assessment of nutrition

For practical clinical purposes a simple assessment of an individual old person's diet may be made by asking questions about how many properly prepared meals are available each week and by asking patients to give a broad description of the types of food, and amounts, in their diet. More precise assessments can be made by recruiting the help of a dietician, and this is particularly useful if there is obvious clinical evidence of subnutrition or overnutrition.

Management

The vast majority of elderly people will maintain adequate nutrition without special arrangements being made; families and friends are often very supportive and a surprising number of elderly people, even those living alone, prepare adequate food themselves. If nutritional status is thought to be precarious, the following measures will often provide sufficient supplementation:

- 'Meals-on-wheels', who provide 1 properly prepared meal per day (5 per week is often enough)
- multivitamin supplementation for those who insist on an unusual or very restrictive diet
- protein supplements for people who cannot or will not eat natural high-protein foods
- attendance at luncheon clubs, which can provide decent meals as well as an opportunity to socialize.

There is some debate as to whether vitamin supplementation should be given routinely. While there is no doubt that small groups of old people have inadequate vitamin intake, there does not seem to be any justification for the wholesale vitamin supplementation of old people's diets. Evidence of diseases such as osteomalacia and scurvy clearly indicates the need for supplementation. There is also a good case to be made for vitamin supplementation for people who are included in the high-risk groups defined above. Supplementation should be with the water-soluble vitamins (B group and C) and vitamin D.

Nutritional needs are directly related to the expenditure of energy. In old age this is diminished in a number of ways. Increased disability leads to decreased exercise; retirement also causes diminished energy expenditure. However, in modern society automation has removed the very high energy expenditure from many forms of occupation. The use of motorized transport also reduces energy utilization. The important point to remember is that overall energy intake needs to match energy expenditure in a person of any age maintaining a steady body weight.

Additional calorie intake may be required for a period of time in the recovery phase from a severe acute illness while weight is being regained.

Nutritional support during acute severe illnesses

Recent research has shown that elderly patients are particularly vulnerable to subnutrition when being treated in hospital for acute severe medical and surgical illnesses. The patients often have high energy requirements at such times because of, for example, fever, a raised respiratory and heart rate and wound healing. However, it is not unusual for a patient to go virtually without food or any form of nutrition for several days.

Not only is it likely that this impairs recovery from the acute illness but it is also probable that subsequent rehabilitation is impaired by protein and calorie malnutrition in such people. A detailed consideration of nutritional support can be found in specialized textbooks. However, the measures listed in Box 19.2 are recommended as good practice to minimize subnutrition in acutely ill elderly people.

Box 19.2 Measures to minimize subnutrition

- If the patient is able to take food by mouth, encouragement should be given to take small, frequent, appetizing meals.
- Intravenous fluid regimens should include, when appropriate, dextrose-containing fluids.
- Patients unable to swallow after, for example, stroke should receive nutritional support through a fine-bore nasogastric tube, not later than the third day of the illness.
- Patients with stroke or other neurological lesions leading to longer-term inability to swallow should have a per-endoscopic gastrostomy tube placed before severe subnutrition is present.
- Patients unable to take enteral nutrition but who are likely to recover from, for example, a surgical operation, should receive balanced parenteral nutrition through a centrally placed venous line, beginning early in the recovery phase.
- Care must be taken to correct any vitamin or trace element deficiencies.

Obesity

Changes in the disposition of fat stores seem to occur in human beings as they age, with movement of fat from subcutaneous tissues to deep tissues, and from the limbs to the trunk. Generally speaking, very obese people do not survive into old age. Those who do are not found to have a higher calorie intake than a non-obese person and have often had a stable weight for many years.

It is assumed that at some stage in life they have consumed more calories than they utilized with obesity as the result. Aged obese people are usually physically inactive, which further reduces their ability to burn up their fat stores. Elderly obese people are more likely to be hypertensive, diabetic and have problems with osteoarthrotic joints. They are less likely to be mobile than their lean counterparts. However, attempts to achieve weight reduction are very rarely successful. An obese elderly person requires severe calorie restriction over a long period of time to lose significant amounts of weight, and this runs the risk of causing deficiency of other nutrients. Few elderly people are prepared to embark upon such a regimen unless some very strong motivating factor is present.

Peripheral vascular disease and musculoskeletal disease

Introduction

In this chapter it is intended to deal with a number of clinical conditions which, while common or with their maximal incidence in advanced age, nevertheless are well recognized by physicians and surgeons and adequately dealt with in textbooks of medicine and surgery. It is not intended, therefore, to deal with them extensively, but simply to bring out those points which are of particular importance in old age.

Vascular disease

Peripheral arterial disease

Atherosclerosis is the basic pathological condition underlying a great deal of morbidity in elderly people, and one of its most important effects is to produce the ischaemic foot. This usually presents clinically in one of four ways:

- pain alone, either intermittent claudication occurring in the calf on exercise, or rest pain in the foot, often confined to the heel, and often occurring during the night
- pre-gangrene, which presents as discoloration of part of the extremity of the foot, usually but not always associated with pain
- gangrene with discoloration associated with coldness and usually with pain in the early stages, though it may be pain-free once fully established
- bacterial infection, which often complicates gangrene and pre-gangrene, particularly around the nails or between the toes.

Clinical assessment and management

Inspection of the feet with palpation of the peripheral pulses should be a routine part of every physical examination in old people, and in peripheral arterial disease a careful note must be taken of the presence and nature of the arterial pulses in the groin and the popliteal fossa as well as the posterior tibial and dorsalis pedis pulses.

Additional information about the peripheral circulation can be obtained by the following methods:

- Ultrasound estimation of blood flow through the peripheral arteries: is a useful semiquantitative method which gives information about blood flow in the main vessel.
- Contrast arteriography will outline the arterial circulation in detail, but should only be carried out if it is intended to proceed to vascular surgery should an operable arterial obstruction be discovered.

General measures. The following general measures are important in all people with peripheral vascular disease, irrespective of whether or not they will proceed to surgery:

- Smokers should try to stop; this is probably the single most important measure they can take to improve their peripheral circulation and reduce the risk of gangrene.

- Patients with diabetes should have their condition controlled as well as possible, and infection should be looked for and treated vigorously.
- Exercise has been shown to be beneficial in patients with intermittent claudication, largely by encouraging the development of collateral blood supply to the lower limbs. Obviously, this is not a suitable treatment for patients with pre-gangrene or gangrene.
- The use of vasodilator drugs remains controversial. However, some patients appear to benefit symptomatically when treated with drugs such as cyclandelate or naftidrofuryl, though these drugs should not be given continually if there is no benefit after about 4 weeks.

Surgical treatment. A proportion of patients will require surgical treatment, including the following measures:

- Patients with intermittent claudication or rest pain who have surgically remediable obstructions in the arterial supply to the leg can benefit from bypass grafting.
- Patients with an acutely obstructive artery due to thromboembolism can have a limb salvaged by performing embolectomy.
- Patients with peripheral gangrene, pre-gangrene or severe intractable ischaemic pain sometimes require amputation.
- The peripheral circulation in some patients can be improved by performing a semipermanent lumbar sympathetic ganglion block using an injection of diluted phenol.

Details of the management of an ischaemic foot can be found in surgical textbooks, and it is very important that patients with critically ischaemic feet have an early consultation with a surgeon so that the full range of surgical therapies can be considered. After amputation patients will require full structured rehabilitation in a specialist geriatric rehabilitation department, and many are able to wear and use a limb prosthesis.

Venous thrombosis

Venous thrombosis is an important and common condition in elderly people, and the various risk factors for venous thrombosis become increasingly prevalent with age.

The most important risk factors can be summarized as follows:

- immobility from any cause, which leads to venous stasis in the lower limbs
- injury to the lower limbs, either accidental or surgical; there is a very high incidence of deep venous thrombosis in people after traumatic or elective hip surgery
- stroke, partly because of the immobility, though the affected limb is particularly vulnerable to deep venous thrombosis
- congestive cardiac failure
- incompetent deep vein valves and varicose veins
- underlying pathological conditions causing a prothrombotic state, such as carcinoma, sepsis or polycythaemia
- rare prothrombotic states such as antithrombin 3 deficiency and deficiency in protein S and protein C, though these usually manifest earlier in life.

Superficial thrombophlebitis manifests itself as redness and pain limited to part of the calf, and the affected vein is tender. It is usually treated by firm binding of the leg, analgesics and restricted activity but not complete rest. Recurrent episodes of superficial thrombophlebitis (thrombophlebitis migrans) are sometimes an early sign of an unsuspected malignancy.

Deep venous thrombosis is particularly important in the elderly, especially in those who are immobilized, for example, as a result of a stroke, or those undergoing pelvic surgery or surgery of the hip joint.

Its special importance lies in the fact that it predisposes to pulmonary embolism, a not uncommon cause of death in old people. The other long-term complication of deep venous thrombosis is peripheral stasis with the production of leg ulcers.

Deep vein thrombosis can present in a number of ways:

- It may be asymptomatic and insidious and present with a pulmonary embolism.
- There may be gradual swelling of the calf with minimal tenderness.

- It may present as an acute illness with rapid swelling of the lower limb, pain, particularly on dorsiflexion of the affected foot, and diversion of blood flow to the superficial veins.

Investigation

In a typical case the diagnosis is often obvious, but in the more insidious case there can be considerable doubt. It is also known that some deep venous thromboses are completely asymptomatic and will only be detected by routine screening. The following investigations can be of practical help:

- Ultrasound sonovenography is a helpful, noninvasive method of detecting deep venous thrombosis, particularly in the upper part of the leg. This enables the clinician to screen out the thromboses which are more likely to be of clinical significance and with a higher risk of pulmonary embolism. The technique is less good for demonstrating venous thrombosis below the knee.
- The most accurate method is contrast venography which can be used to outline the venous drainage of the whole limb, with a high degree of reliability and specificity.
- Gamma camera scans of the limbs after injection of radioactive iodine-labelled fibrinogen is another useful method which produces few false positive and false negative results, though it is less accurate than venography.

If involvement of the pelvic veins and inferior vena cava is suspected this can be confirmed by performing an abdominal and pelvic computed tomography (CT) scan.

Prevention of deep venous thrombosis

Prevention of deep venous thrombosis is extremely important. All elderly people lying in bed should be encouraged to keep their legs moving, and those who are very immobile, particularly when a pro thrombotic condition is present such as pneumonia or septicaemia, should receive low-dose subcutaneous heparin prophylaxis. Surgical departments should also be encouraged to use techniques peri-operatively which reduce the risk of deep venous thrombosis, including the use of heparin in some cases, careful positioning of limbs, and the use of mechanical intermittent compression devices of the lower limbs during prolonged operations.

Treatment of deep venous thrombosis

If the diagnosis of deep venous thrombosis has been proven, or there is a strong clinical suspicion, the treatment consists of a number of elements:

- There should be initial anticoagulation with heparin, unless there is a contraindication.
- The affected limb should be elevated.
- Analgesia to control pain should be given. Nonsteroidal anti-inflammatory drugs such as ibuprofen and diclofenac are very effective but need to be used carefully in patients who are anticoagulated; paracetamol is often sufficient.
- As soon as the limb is reasonably comfortable, patients should be encouraged to start weight-bearing and walking around.

In patients with a deep venous thrombosis due to a predisposing cause which has been removed, 8 weeks of anticoagulation with warfarin is usually sufficient; the patient is transferred from heparin to warfarin whilst still an inpatient. Patients who have had apparently idiopathic deep venous thromboses may have underlying serious pathology for which there should be a careful search. For example, elderly men should be examined and investigated for evidence of carcinoma of the prostate and many clinicians organize abdominal and pelvic ultrasound scans to rule out masses which might predispose to lower limb thrombosis.

In patients who cannot be given long-term warfarin therapy because of contraindications or risk factors, a reasonable compromise is to apply a lower limb compression stocking, encourage mobility and try to minimize any predisposing risk factors for thrombosis.

The role of aspirin as an anticoagulant in this context is controversial; there should be a benefit theoretically, but this has not been proven conclusively in clinical trials. The same applies to other drugs with anticoagulant properties such as hydroxychloroquine and dipyridamole.

Chronic leg ulcers

Chronic leg ulcers are a common and sometimes intractable problem in elderly people. They usually occur in the lower third of the calf or around the ankle, may be single or multiple, painful or asymptomatic, and are associated generally with venous stasis, either after deep vein thrombosis or in association with immobility, postural oedema of the legs and varicose veins.

Such ulcers are sometimes referred to as chronic venous ulcers, though the differential diagnosis includes several other conditions which are outlined in Box 20.1; the clinician must take care to make an accurate diagnosis in such cases.

Box 20.1 Causes of lower limb ulceration in old age

- Venous stasis ulcers
- True arterial ulcers
- Mixed ulcers due to venous and arterial insufficiency.
- Pyoderma gangrenosum
- Cellulitis due to bacterial infection with secondary ulceration
- In the tropics, the various causes of tropical ulcers

Management involves treatment of any superficial infection or cellulitis. Topical treatment is usually adequate, and systemic antibiotics are only indicated if there is an appreciable surrounding area of cellulitis. Necrotic tissue needs to be removed and abscesses need to be drained. Most chronic leg ulcers will eventually heal with a combination of bed rest, elevation of the limb and non-weight-bearing active exercises. The healing process is slow and care must be taken to avoid other attendant risks of a period of immobility and bed rest. Daily physiotherapy is essential. Unfortunately, many leg ulcers relapse either as a result of minor trauma or because of recurring postural oedema in patients who remain chairfast, and patients who sleep in a chair are particularly at risk. Elastic stockings should therefore be provided as soon as the ulcers have healed, though these should be used with great care if there is evidence of arterial insufficiency. Some patients benefit from arterial bypass grafting if an ischaemic component is contributing to the ulcer, and in some patients healing of a large ulcer can be speeded up by split skin grafting once granulation tissue has formed.

Joint disease in elderly patients

Osteoarthrosis

Age-associated change in synovial joints is extremely common even from early adult life and these changes are similar to those seen in osteoarthrosis. There is not a full understanding of whether such changes are always pathological or whether they are sometimes simply due to wear and tear with advancing age. The changes of osteoarthrosis include:

- unevenness of the articular surface
- fibrillation and formation of clefts and fissures in the cartilage matrix
- the erosion of hyaline cartilage with consequent eburnation of the bone
- cyst formation in the subchondral marrow spaces.

Such changes may be regarded as pathological when they are associated with additional factors which add to the trauma and stress experienced particularly by the large weight-bearing joints, in which case the condition is referred to as secondary osteoarthrosis. In such patients one or more joints are affected, usually in an asymmetrical manner, often with considerable deformity and pain.

Secondary osteoarthrosis may be seen in patients with obesity, previous joint diseases – for example, Perthe's disease in childhood, previous fracture and in certain occupational groups who traumatize their joints such as footballers, workers in heavy manual jobs and those who use heavy vibrating machinery. A condition sometimes referred to as primary generalized osteoarthrosis is seen in the absence of such risk factors and is most common in postmenopausal women. It produces a symmetrical arthrosis affecting particularly the distal interphalangeal joints and first carpo-metacarpal joints, but also may affect other joints including the apophyseal joints of the spine.

This condition has a slow onset in most cases but can occur subacutely; the general course is benign, the appearance of the hands is characterized by the formation of Heberden's nodes, and the hands usually remain dextrous and useful. Primary generalized osteoarthrosis almost certainly has an important genetic component in its pathogenesis, and this contention is supported by the fact that the condition tends to run in families and is commoner in Caucasians than in other races.

Acute exacerbation of osteoarthrosis

Sometimes an osteoarthrotic joint becomes acutely painful, swollen and hot. In a substantial proportion of such patients the acute deterioration is caused by a crystal arthropathy due to the presence of hydroxyapatite crystals in the synovial space. Such crystals cannot be seen by light microscopy but are detected by the electron microscope. The condition settles with rest and antiflammatory therapy. Of course, in a patient with an acutely inflamed osteoarthrotic joint, care must be taken to rule out the other possible causes of acute arthritis which are listed below.

Rheumatoid arthritis

Rheumatoid arthritis can start acutely in advanced old age, or patients may grow old with it in a burnt-out form from earlier life. Acute rheumatoid arthritis in old age is often atypical and may show a very aggressive onset, often involving the larger joints in the early stages. Rheumatoid arthritis in elderly people often responds very well to modest doses of corticosteroid therapy, and the joints often settle down quickly and remain quiescent. The coexistence of chronic rheumatoid arthritis and osteoarthrosis sometimes poses diagnostic difficulties in the elderly. Rheumatoid involvement in the hands is generally in the proximal interphalangeal joints as well as the metacarpo-phalangeal and wrist joints, whereas osteoarthrosis affects the distal interphalangeal joints. Radiographs of the hands often enable a distinction to be made in uncertain cases.

Serological tests to help support the diagnosis of rheumatoid arthritis in elderly people can be performed along the same lines as in the younger person.

A proportion of the patients will have IgM rheumatoid factor, and in an acute case, the erythrocyte sedimentation rate (ESR) and C-reactive protein (CRP) levels will be high.

Acute monarticular arthritis in elderly people

In geriatric medicine it is common to encounter an elderly person with a single inflamed joint. The important features of acute arthritis are:

- pain and stiffness
- peri-articular swelling, often with a joint effusion
- redness and heat of the affected joint.

There are a number of conditions which must be considered in a patient presenting in this way, and it is important to distinguish one from another as different treatments are required:

- *Monarticular rheumatoid arthritis.* This is a variant of rheumatoid arthritis which is commoner in old people than in the young. The onset is usually subacute, serological markers for rheumatoid arthritis are sometimes positive, the ESR and CRP levels are high, and aspiration of joint fluid will reveal a sterile effusion without the presence of crystals. Monarticular rheumatoid responds very well to corticosteroid therapy.
- *Crystal arthropathy.* This is usually due to the presence of pyrophosphate crystals causing pseudogout, or uric acid crystals causing gout.

The onset is usually very acute with severe pain. The systemic upset is less than with monarticular rheumatoid or septic arthritis and the ESR and CRP levels may be normal or only moderately raised. Diagnostic confirmation is by aspiration of joint fluid and examination under polarized light for the detection of pyrophosphate or uric acid crystals. Some patients with acute inflammatory flair-ups of osteoarthrosis have a crystal arthropathy caused by hydroxyapatite crystals, though these cannot be seen through a light microscope. Crystal arthropathies respond well to nonsteroidal antiinflammatory drugs, and in the case of gout the patient should have a serum uric acid estimation performed to detect hyperuricaemia, and may require investigations to determine the reason for the high uric acid level, such as malignancy and renal impairment. Diuretic therapy sometimes precipitates gout.

- *Septic arthritis.* This may present as a monarthritis or with several joints involved. The cause is bacterial infection of the joint space and the onset is usually fairly rapid with considerable system upset including fever, malaise and a poor appetite. The patient usually has other evidence of infection, such as a high blood white cell count, rising ESR, persistent fever and high CRP. Confirmation of the diagnosis is made by joint aspiration which will reveal the presence of large numbers of pus cells in the joint fluid, and it is usually possible to stain and culture the infecting bacteria. Treatment is by antibiotic therapy and analgesics. Resting the joint is extremely important in septic arthritis to prevent damage to the joint surface.

There are other rarer causes of monarthritis in the elderly and the student is referred to textbooks of general medicine and rheumatology for more details on these.

It is important to strike a balance between resting the joint during the acute phase and the need to avoid prolonged immobility in an elderly patient. It is usual to start mobilizing the patient as soon as the acute pain has settled, though it is usually advisable to keep a septic joint immobile and non-weight-bearing until it has completely settled.

Foot disorders

Deformities of the feet become increasingly common with advancing age, especially in women. Some of the most important ones encountered are as follows:

- *Corns.* These are discrete, hard, keratinized epithelial plugs which develop over prominent bony points exposed to trauma. They are often associated with hammer toes.
- *Callosities.* These are larger areas of cornified epithelium on the sole of the foot.
- *Bunions.* These are tender and inflamed areas overlying the exostoses which develop at the metacarpal head in patients with hallux valgus.
- *Onychogryphosis.* This is the end result of neglected abnormal thickening of toenails. A hard and curved horn develops. Lesser degrees of thickening are very common and make toenail cutting by normal means impossible.
- *Diabetic foot disorders.* These are dealt with in the chapter on diabetes mellitus.

In all the above conditions treatment by a chiropodist is required. Apart from direct removal of abnormal tissues, chiropodists may provide splints and special footwear to overcome deformities. Toenail cutting in old people with peripheral vascular insufficiency is also best left to the chiropodist. Painful feet are an underestimated cause of poor mobility in elderly patients, so every effort should be made to render the feet comfortable and to provide the necessary adapted footwear.

Part 4

Services for the elderly

21

Rehabilitation

Introduction

The principles of rehabilitation form one of the most important aspects of geriatric medical practice. Many definitions of rehabilitation are seen, though a widely accepted one is: 'restoration of the individual to his or her fullest physical, mental and social capability'.

The emphasis is on treating the patient as a whole rather than focusing on pathological conditions. Ideally, the aim is to obtain the fullest possible recovery, though this is often modified in real clinical practice to obtain the optimum level of improvement needed to restore the individual to independence, and enable him or her to live at home or in residential care.

In many countries, such as the United Kingdom, geriatricians no longer provide long-term custodial care in a hospital setting. Therefore the focus of their work has changed to one of early assessment and active rehabilitation of all suitable aged patients.

Furthermore, since geriatricians in many countries treat very ill elderly patients through their acute illnesses, a large number of frail elderly patients survive longer and accumulate an unpredictable mix of pathological and degenerative conditions. This has resulted in a great need for rehabilitation in such countries to increase the speed of the return of such people to independence and to reduce both morbidity and mortality during that period.

Impairment, disability and handicap

These terms often become confused, so it is worth spending time getting to grips with their meaning.

Impairment. This means an objective reduction from normality in the physical or mental ability of the individual due to disease or disorder which may be temporary or permanent.

Disability. This is the apparent affect that impairment has upon daily function, when subjective differences in adaptation are balanced against normal expected activity.

Handicap. This is the perceived disadvantage within society that results directly from a particular impairment or disability.

It follows, therefore, that the purpose of rehabilitation is to reduce the amount of handicap and disability that results from any particular impairment in an individual.

Recovery. This means a partial or complete return to the premorbid condition. Strictly speaking, this term should be restricted to natural recovery such as that seen spontaneously after a stroke.

It should then be distinguished from the improvements which can be obtained by retraining and adaptation during the process of rehabilitation.

Activities of daily living (ADL)

These are the functional abilities a person needs to be able to live with minimal dependence. They include being able to dress, wash, feed, walk and use the toilet. There are various scales used to assess ADL, one of the most useful of which is the Barthel index shown in Table 21.1.

The multidisciplinary rehabilitation team

Rehabilitation of the elderly is normally coordinated by a clinician with a special interest in geri-

Table 21.1 The Barthel ADL index.

Date

Bowels
0 = incontinent
1 = occasional accident
2 = continent

Bladder
0 = incontinent or catheterized and unable to
    manage
1 = occasional accident (max. 1 × per 24 hours)
2 = continent (for over 7 days)

Grooming
0 = needs help
1 = independent face/hair/teeth/shaving

Toilet use
0 = dependent
1 = needs some help, but can do something
2 = independent (on and off, dressing, wiping)

Feeding
0 = unable
1 = needs help cutting, spreading butter etc.
2 = independent

Transfer
0 = unable
1 = major help (1–2 people, physical)
2 = minor help (verbal or physical)
3 = independent

Mobility
0 = immobile
1 = wheelchair-independent including corners etc.
2 = walks with help of one person (verbal or
    physical)
3 = independent (but may use any aid, e.g. stick)

Dressing
0 = dependent
1 = needs help, but can do about half unaided
2 = dependent

Stairs
0 = unable
1 = needs help (verbal, physical, carrying aid)
2 = independent up and down

Bathing
0 = dependent
1 = independent
TOTAL

atric medicine. Nursing staff with training in nursing the elderly are a vital link in the entire process. The team also comprises physiotherapists and occupational therapists, and there should be close contact with a medical social worker, speech therapist, chiropodist and continence adviser.

Occasionally members have to be coopted into the team for special cases; examples would be a dietician or an expert in pressure sore management.

Where should rehabilitation take place?

It is possible to perform rehabilitation in a wide variety of settings, although the usual arrangement is to have a specially dedicated unit. Rehabilitation wards, often on the site of a general hospital, have been developed by most health authorities in the United Kingdom, and similar facilities are available in other parts of the world, such as Scandinavia, Canada, Australasia and the United States.

Adequate space should be provided around beds and in the bathrooms for hoists and walking aids, both to encourage independence with mobility and to facilitate nursing. Special beds, such as the King's Fund Mark Five, should be available to reduce complications from immobility. Chairs and beds should be of the correct height to aid standing and there should be special showers and baths to aid washing, for both assisted and independent patients. Usually, some single bedrooms are provided and there is an obvious need for a large day room to allow different activities, as well as a secluded room for interviewing patients and relatives.

The physiotherapy gym and occupational therapy department, including a kitchen and bedroom for ADL assessment, should be in close proximity. Ideally, there should be a level outside area such as a garden or patio for use in good weather. The environment should be homely and not too clinical. Some hospitals have also developed dedicated units for specialist rehabilitation. Of particular importance are orthogeriatric rehabilitation wards and stroke units. These specialized units allow the staff with particular skills and specialist interests to be concentrated in one place and also allow closer cooperation between clinicians of different specialties in managing complex cases.

Which patients require rehabilitation?

There is no strict age limit but most patients will be over the age of 65; in a typical rehabilitation ward in the United Kingdom the median age would be around 80 years. There are usually substantially more female patients than male. The majority of patients enter the rehabilitation unit after recovery from an acute illness or combination of illnesses, having originally been under the care of the geriatrician or general physician.

The remainder are either referrals from other medical or surgical specialties after acute admission or are admitted directly to the unit after assessment in the outpatient clinic or in the community by the geriatrician or general practitioner.

Patients vary considerably in their capacity to benefit from rehabilitation, but there is also a variation in the ADL performance of an individual in different settings. For example, a patient who is independent in the hospital environment may behave differently at home and apparently regress when interacting with normal carers and family, even though the carer's demands are well within the patient's capability. Conversely, aged patients with mild cognitive impairment may appear unable to cope when assessed in strange hospital surroundings, but be independent and safe in their own environment.

This variation in performance, combined with factors associated with pathology, ageing, environment and personality, is one of the challenges of geriatric rehabilitation and must be taken into account when planning treatment, discharge and follow-up.

Some patients who are extremely frail as a consequence of being very aged and having multiple disabilities often do less well in formal intensive rehabilitation settings. For this reason, a range of settings for rehabilitation is desirable and ideally will include a slower-stream facility where a greater degree of nursing support is possible. This often takes place in wards also used for continuing care or respite admissions.

Before patients are placed in a rehabilitation set-

ting it is important that some form of assessment is made. For some patients, formal rehabilitation may be inappropriate or even impossible. More stringent entry criteria are often necessary with specialized units, such as orthogeriatric or stroke units, and these often have very specific operational policies, including tightly defined selection criteria.

The process of rehabilitation

Rehabilitation is quite difficult to define. It is not a treatment that can be applied to patients in the same way as, for example, a surgical operation or giving antibiotics for infection.

The entire process builds up on a natural recovery taking place in a patient after an acute illness, and makes the most of remaining function by improving mobility, optimizing medical treatment and helping the patient to reach the highest functional level possible. Rehabilitation also has an important psychological function in building the patient's confidence, reducing anxiety and lifting depression.

Discharge planning

Ideally, discharge planning begins at the time of admission, though detailed plans often have to be left until the patient's functional status is better understood. Discharge preparations should be fine-tuned by regular case review and after full discussion with the patients, carers, social services and district nurses. This prevents unnecessary re-admission and is of obvious benefit to the patient.

However, some discharges are bound to fail because the patients or relatives insist on a discharge against professional advice and hence return to an environment unsuitable for the patient's limited degree of functional independence. The back-up of continued rehabilitation through facilities such as a day hospital or community services, leading to a cushioned discharge, is particularly useful for frailer patients.

At the time of discharge, clear plans and clear methods of communication with the other agencies are essential. The best time for discharge in an individual patient has to be assessed in a bespoke manner, taking into account all relevant details pertaining to that person. Discharge should be considered either when a functional plateau has been reached and further improvements are unlikely; or when functional targets have been reached; or when further rehabilitation can be undertaken in the community, either by community agencies or in a day hospital. It is essential that the rehabilitation team communicates widely with the patient, carers, general practitioner and community agencies or charities who are likely to be involved after discharge.

Day hospitals

An extensive account of day hospitals is given in Chapter 22.

22

Geriatric services

Introduction

In the United Kingdom the geriatric service remains a large and important part of the National Health Service, despite many recent changes in the way it is organized. The service is largely hospital-based and is run and supervised by consultant physicians with a special interest in geriatric medicine. In most parts of the country the centre point of the geriatric service is a district general hospital, serving the local population. The catchment areas are less well defined than they used to be and depend on local agreements with purchasing health authorities and general practice fundholders, though for most geriatric services, catchment areas correspond roughly to health districts. Broadly speaking, the practice of geriatric medicine is based on the general medical model, and in many parts of the United Kingdom, the overwhelming majority of medical emergencies are seen in frail old people, in which case the practice of general medicine and acute geriatric medicine becomes synonymous.

Nevertheless, a proportion of such emergency admissions will consist of patients with the characteristic problems encountered in geriatric medicine, such as confusion, falls and incontinence, in which case there is a need for a strong and well-organized geriatric service to run as part of or alongside the general medical service. As well as acute medical emergencies in frail old people, the geriatric service is charged with the responsibility of organizing rehabilitation and helping to select people for long-term care in nursing homes. Many services also include a day hospital and organize, in conjunction with general practitioners, screening programmes to detect unreported illness and maintain close liaison with community services and voluntary services.

Definition

It is not easy to produce a definition of geriatric medicine which will be acceptable to all geriatricians.

It is basically an organizational rather than age-related specialty, yet in some areas it is practised as an age-related specialty based on the lower age of 70 or 75 years; more often, however, it is based on individual patients' needs, or acutely ill elderly people are admitted to hospital in the first instance as part of an all-age general medical service.

Perhaps the best definition is that proposed by the British Geriatric Society, which is simple yet comprehensible: 'Geriatrics is the branch of general medicine concerned with the clinical, preventive, remedial and social aspects of illness in elderly people.'

The structure of the service

As mentioned above, the service is usually wholly or partly based in a district general hospital, though in many parts of the country, smaller community hospitals are also involved, particularly for rehabilitation.

In most parts of Britain there is also a close working relationship with social services and private sector nursing homes and rest homes who provide the lion's share of continuing care in the community. Broadly speaking, the models of service outlined in Figure 22.1 represent the most common patterns in the United Kingdom. In other

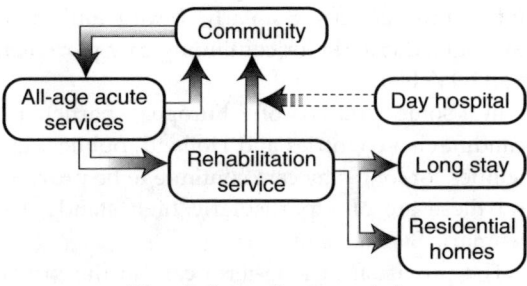

The integrated model

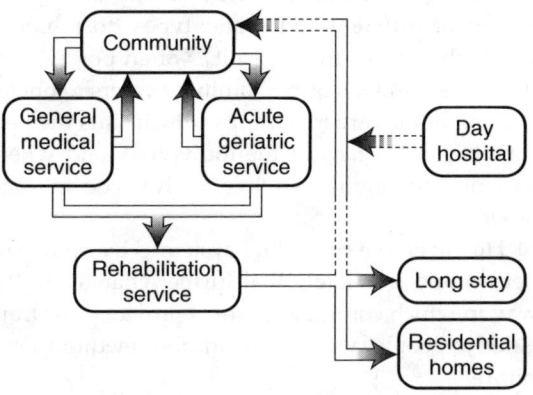

Separate acute geriatric service

Fig. 22.1 Main models of geriatric service in the UK.

parts of the world geriatric services have evolved to meet local requirements, though they often reflect to a certain extent the prevailing structure in the United Kingdom.

Geriatricians usually organize the beds under their care to provide a system of progressive patient care involving stages of acute treatment, rehabilitation and then follow-up after discharge to home, rest home or nursing home with involvement when necessary of the day hospital. Before the early 1980s the NHS also provided a very large number of continuing care beds, though very few services now retain large amounts of continuing care capacity. However, most geriatric services find that they require a small number of continuing care beds for patients who are terminally ill or who require, for medical or nursing reasons, the higher level of technological support that can be provided

in hospital and which cannot be provided by even the best private sector nursing homes.

Acute wards

Acutely ill elderly people are usually admitted to general medical wards (this is particularly appropriate in districts where the majority of medical admissions are of frail elderly patients) or to acute geriatric wards. In either case it is essential to have nursing staff who are sensitive to and trained in dealing with the problems of acutely ill, frail, elderly people.

In such a ward, the initial investigation, treatment and assessment is carried out with the use of whatever ancillary services are required so that a complete series of diagnoses may be made, appropriate medical treatment instigated, and the patient's future care considered.

The length of stay in such a ward varies in different parts of the country, largely depending upon the availability and type of facilities available for the next stage of management. In most parts of Britain, the average length of stay in the acute ward would be between 5 and 15 days.

From the acute ward a large proportion of elderly patients will go home or return to their rest home or nursing home. Some will die and others will proceed to rehabilitation.

Rehabilitation ward

Rehabilitation wards are usually situated in the general hospital or in an affiliated community hospital. Patients are generally transferred to the rehabilitation ward from acute wards, or may be transferred directly from another inpatient facility, or after assessment in the outpatient clinic, day hospital or at home.

Patients requiring rehabilitation are predominantly those suffering from stroke, parkinsonism, arthritis, fractures and amputations, and the generalized weakness which often follows an acute medical illness in old age. Of course, the whole spectrum of disabling disease can be dealt with in a rehabilitation ward. Some rehabilitation wards become specialized, particularly those dealing with stroke rehabilitation, which are often part of formal stroke units, and those providing rehabilitation for patients recovering from orthopaedic trauma, particularly fracture of the neck of the femur.

The average length of stay varies enormously between individual patients and departments, and often depends on the availability and sophistication of follow-up services in the community. In the author's hospital, the average length for general geriatric rehabilitation is 16 days, and 25 and 28 days for the stroke unit and orthogeriatric units respectively.

At the end of that time the larger number of patients will return to their own homes or to the residential home from which they originated. Some will have died and a small number will remain so disabled that they require placement in a nursing home; some who are medically unstable or terminally ill may be transferred to an NHS continuing care unit.

Long-term care

This aspect of the geriatric service has changed radically in recent years in Britain, and has now come to resemble the model prevalent in parts of the United States of America. The main change has been the dramatic reduction in size and scale of long-term care provision within the NHS and the rapid growth of nursing home and rest home provision by the private sector. Such private sector facilities are subject to certain quality standards, and nursing homes are monitored and licensed by health authorities whilst rest homes are regulated by social services departments. However, most geriatric services retain a small number of continuing care beds for patients who are too ill to be discharged to the private sector.

Patients requiring a private sector nursing home need nursing care and in most cases they are likely to remain in nursing home care for the rest of their lives. Patients whose total assets fall below a certain threshold will have their rest home or nursing home fees paid by social services departments.

Therefore, social services staff need to be involved in the assessment of patients for placement in such facilities, and in most districts in the United Kingdom, the criteria for such placements have been broadly agreed between social services

and health services. Similarly, health authorities have agreed criteria for continuing care placement in an NHS bed.

In some parts of Europe, particularly Scandinavian countries and Holland, public sector facilities for long-stay care continue to be provided and these are of a particularly high standard in Denmark, Sweden and Norway.

The provision of long-term care in the private sector has been criticized on the grounds that commercial motivation may lead to an inferior service.

On the other hand, a wide variety of nursing homes of different styles and types does give a wider choice to patients, so it is often possible for the patient and his or her family or carers to obtain nursing home care in a facility which suits the personality and means of the individual, and where patient and family can live fairly close to each other.

However, the prevailing system is by no means perfect and it is likely that further changes to the way in which continuing care is provided for frail, elderly people will occur in the medium-term future.

Hospital continuing care wards require nursing staff who are dedicated to the care of very frail elderly people, many of whom will be unable to communicate and all of whom will require help with virtually all physical activities. Some nurses choose to specialize in this type of care, and since the ambience on the ward needs to be quite different from that in a rehabilitation ward, a strong case can be made for having continuing care facilities separate from those where active treatment is taking place.

In parts of the country with extensive nursing home provision the patients who remain for continuing care are so frail that their average life expectancy is usually less than 3 months, though some do live much longer than that.

Holiday and respite admissions

Many departments of geriatric medicine reserve one or two beds, often in a continuing care ward, to admit patients who are being nursed at home by their relatives, on a short-term prearranged admission, to allow the relatives to have a holiday or rest.

Care of a disabled old person at home, particularly if there is some mental impairment, is a demanding and unremitting responsibility. Unless those who carry it out can obtain relief from time to time it is likely that the situation will eventually break down and some form of long-term care will be sought for the old person. Holiday admission is a method of trying to prevent such breakdown. Hospital admission is only necessary when special skills or equipment are required, and a large proportion of respite admissions take place in private sector nursing homes. Occasionally, respite admission can be combined with rehabilitation to help keep a frail old person reasonably mobile.

The geriatric day hospital

Day hospitals form an important part of the overall service by providing an extension of progressive care, beyond the period of inpatient treatment.

They allow the patient to have the benefit of hospital investigation and treatment whilst still able to live at home. They are thus both an advantage to patients and economic of staff. Generally speaking, patients attend the day hospital for four reasons:

- rehabilitation
- maintenance treatment
- further assessment and monitoring of social needs
- medical and nursing investigation and treatment.

Patients with apparently similar diagnoses may attend for any one or combination of these purposes, so it is extremely important that the geriatrician and all the staff should be aware of the reasons why each patient is attending, and regular case conferences to discuss progress are needed.

Day hospital rehabilitation

Prevailing practice in many units driven by the pressure of the large number of patients presenting with acute illnesses is to keep people in rehabilitation wards for as short a time as possible.

Consequently, the day hospital is very useful for rehabilitation to continue after the patient leaves the hospital. Also, rehabilitation may be planned on a day hospital basis without previous admission, if the patient has been assessed in clinic or at home. Rehabilitation envisages improvement and once improvement ceases and the patient reaches the maximum degree of independence then rehabilitation should also be withdrawn. At this stage it is necessary to decide whether the patient's situation and motivation are sufficient to maintain the degree of independence which has been reached or whether further frequent or regular supervision from the hospital to help to maintain this level of independence is required. In such a case the patient will require maintenance attendance or cyclical attendance at the day hospital.

Maintenance treatment at day hospital usually requires less frequent attendance than active rehabilitation: for example, one attendance per week, though this should always be tailored to the patient's individual requirements.

Social assessment and care

Some day hospitals provide social care for patients whose disabilities are so great that they need constant nursing assistance. Such patients attend for three reasons:

- so that they may be cared for each day while relatives go out to work
- so that they may be cared for one day a week to give their relatives a break and to allow the patient an opportunity of socializing and meeting other people
- for social assessment which also entails reviewing the services tending the patient and carers at home and reorganizing them when necessary.

Many day hospitals no longer provide such services, largely because the need is met by social services day centres, since these now often employ some nursing staff. The amount of social care provided by day hospitals will be dictated largely by local requirement and the availability of other local facilities.

Medical and nursing investigations and treatment

The day hospital is a very good setting for the investigation and assessment of certain medical conditions, particularly those where observation of the patient over a substantial period of time leads to the gathering of useful diagnostic information. Examples include Parkinson's disease, disorders of cognitive function, disorders of behaviour, falls and blackouts, and incontinence. Therefore, a modern day hospital will include a wide range of diagnostic activities aimed at refining the diagnosis in patients with these types of problem. Furthermore, day hospitals often incorporate certain types of outpatient clinic, particularly Parkinson's disease clinics and syncope and falls clinics.

The day hospital is also very useful for monitoring patients who are having their drug therapy altered or stabilized, and can be used to carry out certain medical procedures such as sigmoidoscopy, glucose tolerance tests or blood transfusions. The concentration of nursing expertise in day hospitals is also a useful medium for dealing with incontinence, constipation and chronic lower limb ulceration.

Management of the day hospital

The day hospital should be managed in a dynamic way; patients should attend for a limited period of time, being discharged whenever possible. Since discharge often means going back to isolation after having enjoyed a period of socialization, it is often helpful to transfer the patients who no longer need day hospital care to a day centre. Day centres provide social care and indeed many of them provide baths, hairdressing, laundry, chiropody and other services including some nursing, though they do not have the medical and therapeutic staff that a day hospital does.

The medical management of a day hospital is very similar to that of a hospital ward. Day-to-day contact between junior medical staff and patients is essential and there should be a regular round or case conference with the consultant geriatrician.

The psychiatry of old age

The psychiatry of old age, sometimes called psychogeriatrics, is a well-established special branch of psychiatry analogous with child psychiatry.

The psychogeriatrician is a psychiatrist with responsibility for the complete management of the whole range of psychiatric problems in old age. He or she is likely to have a complement of acute beds, a few long-term care beds and a day hospital which form the focus of a multidisciplinary service which has very close links with numerous community agencies and voluntary organizations. In patients with chronic confusional states assessment is made either as an outpatient or inpatient to allow a comprehensive and clear diagnosis to be made of the cause of the confusion, and for this to be managed as far as possible in a community setting.

It is usual to separate facilities for demented patients from those which deal with psychiatric illness, such as depression or acute psychoses in old age, since the management and prognosis are very different and require differing skills. Some patients require long-term NHS care or placement in specialized nursing homes, particularly for the following problems:

- those suffering from chronic brain failure with associated behavioural problems, where it is no longer practical for relatives or other carers to manage the patient at home
- those with chronic brain failure who do not have behavioural problems but have no carers who are willing to take on the responsibility of looking after them in the long term
- those suffering from chronic brain failure who also have severe physical incapacity and require nursing.

Of course, patients with acute brain failure usually have underlying acute medical illnesses and these are usually admitted under the care of the consultant geriatrician as part of an acute general medical or acute geriatric service.

The psychogeriatric day hospital should be separate from, although it may be associated with, the geriatric day hospital. Its primary function is to look after old people suffering from chronic brain failure while their relatives work, or to provide their relatives with some freedom. It also gives an opportunity to obtain optimal management of symptoms and to investigate and treat associated physical disorders.

Psychogeriatrics has now become a large and sophisticated branch of medicine and the student is referred to specialized textbooks for further details. It is important to remember that depressive illnesses in old age can easily be overlooked and are sometimes difficult to diagnose, but have a good prognosis when properly treated. For this reason, the possibility of depression must always be considered in an elderly patient who becomes agitated, negative or withdrawn, and where there is doubt an opinion should be sought from a specialist in psychogeriatric medicine.

The ascertainment of unreported illness

In recent years there have been a number of initiatives in the United Kingdom, some of them national and some local to try to improve the detection of previously unreported illness in elderly people. The need for this was highlighted by studies which showed that about one third of patients suffering from locomotor, respiratory, gastrointestinal, cardiovascular and central nervous system disease had not had the respective problem assessed or diagnosed by their general practitioner.

In Britain the over-75 screening programme has improved things to a certain extent, as has a greater awareness of the need to look for unreported disease in old age and an increasing awareness amongst elderly people themselves and their relatives that early assessment and treatment can improve symptoms and quality of life.

As a problem, unreported illness in old age is unevenly distributed in Britain; for example, there is some evidence to suggest that there is a much higher detection rate of physical ill health in communities with relatively prosperous elderly people, such as the towns of the south coast of England, compared with areas of social and economic deprivation in the large industrial cities and in some remote rural areas. In other parts of the world the detection of illness in elderly people often reflects the prevailing medical culture; for example, prosperous elderly North Americans are known to seek out medical advice and investigation far more actively than their counterparts in most parts of Europe. Also, in countries with weaker economies and a poorer health-care system, recent research has shown that a vast amount of unreported ill health is prevalent in elderly people, with very convincing evidence from Ghana, Gambia, parts of South America and parts of India.

Most previously unreported illness can be detected by taking careful histories and making physical examinations when patients have contact with doctors, and a reasonably high yield can be obtained from certain screening tests, particularly routine urinalysis for protein blood and sugar, full blood count (FBC) to detect anaemia, blood pressure measurement, eye testing and hearing testing. General practitioners, health visitors and practice nurses are best placed to screen large numbers of people in this way, though it is also important to make such screening part and parcel of all hospital consultations.

Geriatric care worldwide

As populations age throughout the world, governments and those responsible for medical care have had to consider how this great challenge to the practice of medicine may best be met. This rapid growth in the population of elderly people is not confined to rich and industrially advanced countries. For example, countries such as Kenya, Zimbabwe, Panama and Indonesia also have a rapidly growing total number of people over the age of 70. Specialist geriatric care, in the medical sense, is most developed in Britain, Holland and the Scandinavian countries.

There are also excellent systems, often based along the same lines as the British model, in parts of Canada, Australia and the United States of America. New Zealand has a rapidly developing geriatric service which now covers most of the country and there are excellent examples of high-quality geriatric practice in Hong Kong and Singapore.

The specialty of geriatric medicine is now much more widely recognized than it was 15 years ago. Most European countries now recognize it in some shape or form, even when the health-care system of such countries does not provide a comprehensive geriatric service.

Throughout the world, universities with medical schools are now recognizing the specialty of geriatric medicine, with or without the scientific discipline of gerontology, and such units are becoming the focus for appropriate planning for the health care of elderly people to suit the prevailing social and economic climate of those countries. For example, there are now departments of geriatric medicine or gerontology in several universities in India, South Africa, Zimbabwe, Ghana, Brazil, Argentina and Peru, and this is by no means an exhaustive list.

It is vital that the pattern of development of geriatric medicine and gerontology reflects local need.

This need will vary according to local patterns of pathology, social structures, availability of finance, the sophistication of national and local government organizations, and the availability of expertise. Geriatric medicine is now seen as one of the major specialties of medicine in Britain, Scandinavia, several other European countries, Australasia and North America and it is likely that this influence will spread in response to need and driven by the enthusiasm of dedicated practitioners and academics in the field.

Voluntary services

Volunteers have always played an important part in Great Britain in making life easier for underprivileged groups, and a great deal of voluntary activity is directed both to old people in their own homes and also to old people in hospital. Many other countries also have a strong voluntary sector, and the way in which volunteers are organized and deployed varies according to the traditions and culture in various parts of the world. In the United Kingdom the major organization concerned with this type of care is Age Concern, which began in 1940 as the National Old People's Welfare Committee but subsequently became the National Old People's Welfare Council. This movement has sponsored the development of local committees in virtually every part of the United Kingdom, each of which in turn has been responsible for the development of old people's clubs, the organization of friendly visitors for isolated old people at home, and in some cases for the provision of 'meals on wheels' and other forms of practical assistance. These are the most important voluntary services provided in the community, but Age Concern organizations undertake to set up a host of other activities, listed in Box 23.1.

Box 23.1 Activities set up by Age Concern Organizations

- The arrangement of holidays for old people
- Help with gardening and house decorating
- The provision of organized good neighbour services
- The provision of day centres and special transport to take old people to them
- Transport to visit their relatives in hospital
- Other services depending on individual needs

In some parts of the United Kingdom, other similar charities such as Help the Aged raise funds for similar types of support. Where the local Age Concern committees are strong, as in many of the counties and larger towns, they act as a coordinating body for all services for the elderly, and representatives of the various voluntary services meet with representatives of hospital geriatric services, social services, housing departments and education departments, to discuss together the needs of old people in their area and particularly the contribution that can be made by volunteer groups.

Age Concern (England) and its counterparts in Scotland, Wales and Northern Ireland are also involved in social action and the promotion of old people's welfare at a national level.

Age Concern has commissioned much research both into its own activities – for example voluntary visiting, day care and special housing for the elderly – and also into the wider needs and aspirations of old people, such as problems with heating, special problems of minority groups such as ageing immigrants, and the rights of old people in institutions.

Age Concern collates information of all types about elderly people and ageing and distributes this widely. It provides training courses for volunteers as well as for workers in various types of health and social care and it speaks for the elderly on a national scale about their needs and problems. Age Concern publishes many reports on these issues.

Voluntary work in hospitals

Many hospitals now employ a full-time coordinator of voluntary services whose responsibility it is to recruit volunteers and to deploy them throughout the hospital in areas where their services are most needed and in work which they will enjoy doing.

Many of these organizers have been extremely successful in their work, which is of particular importance in relation to patients in rehabilitation and continuing care wards in both the geriatric and psychogeriatric services. Another important organization, enjoyed by most hospitals, is the Hospital League of Friends which coordinates a wide range of fund-raising activities to generate money to provide additional facilities, furnishings and fittings over and above those which are the responsibility of the Health Service.

In some parts of the UK, Hospital Leagues of Friends raise very large sums of money which have a major impact on the style and comfort of hospital accommodation for elderly people.

Students are strongly recommended to find out what the voluntary services are in the locality and hospital in which their training is taking place. One of the most effective ways of learning about this aspect of care is to meet with and talk to the hospital volunteers coordinator and, if possible, someone who is a member of the local branch of Age Concern.

Social services

Historical background

There has been some kind of statutory social service in Great Britain since 1601, when the *Poor Relief Act* set the responsibility for the poor and disabled squarely on the shoulders of the local parish. It was laid down that the able-bodied should work, children should be bound apprentice and the halt, the lame, the impotent and the blind should be given relief. Care of the old has ridden on the back of care of the disabled ever since. This system worked reasonably well for more than 200 years, until 1834, when a Board of Guardians was set up to supervise conditions; it adopted the principle of 'less eligibility', which really meant that the 'workhouse' was to be made sufficiently less pleasant than life outside to discourage people from entering it, and so it was. Consequently, reliance on the workhouse came to carry a certain stigma; even now, in the 1990s, some of our very aged patients have such a strong memory of this that some of the present-day hospitals which were originally built as workhouses can still cause them some fear and trepidation.

The *Local Government Act* of 1929 replaced the Boards of Guardians with local and county authorities. The period 1929–1948 was the heyday of the voluntary hospitals and the infirmaries but these concentrated largely on acute medical conditions and bypassed old people except for the chronic sick wards. With the advent of the Health Service in 1948, workhouses were gradually taken over and many of them became hospitals. Furthermore, the *National Assistance Act* of 1948, pioneered by Aneurin Bevan, put a statutory duty on the local authority to provide residential care for old people who could not manage to live at home. Despite many changes in the way such provision is organized, the principle of local authority responsibility for the residential care of frail, old people remains today in the United Kingdom. Other countries have arrangements with parallel or, in some cases, very different histories and students from countries other than the United Kingdom are recommended to find out exactly what the prevailing statutory arrangements are in their country.

The social services in the United Kingdom have steadily increased in both extent and variety since that time and, though they inevitably have limited resources, are of great importance to a large number of old people, many of whom could not survive independently in their own homes without the help offered.

Organization

In the United Kingdom the social services and the health service are independent of one another, though in many districts there is a healthy dialogue between the two services to establish working patterns which are mutually acceptable, and in the general interest of the patients. Social service departments are set up by local authorities, usually county councils, city councils, and more recently, in some parts of the United Kingdom, smaller unitary authorities. The local authorities allocate funds for the maintenance and improvement of services. The actual range of provision depends to a certain extent on the prevailing political balance within the local authority, though in the 1990s there is much less variation in provision across the United Kingdom than was the case 20 years ago.

Social service departments often correspond more or less with health districts or sectors of health districts, though this is not always the case.

The most recent round of reorganizations within the working structure of social service departments, mainly in response to social services legislation in the early 1980s and in 1990, has resulted in the loss of dedicated social workers specializing in the care of the elderly, to be replaced by care managers who are responsible for assessing the need for social services support in individual patients, both in a hospital setting and while the patients are still at home. Money from social services budgets to support frail elderly people cannot be released until this care management assessment process has taken place.

Where old people are concerned, social services departments are responsible for assessing the need for, purchasing and reviewing a range of services. These are listed in Box 24.1.

Box 24.1 Services provided by the social services

- Residential accommodation, often in the private sector, in rest homes or nursing homes, though some districts still retain social services-run old people's homes
- Home help services, sometimes purchased from private home help companies and sometimes provided directly by social services staff
- 'Meals on wheels', usually purchased from private companies, though sometimes provided from kitchens run by social services departments and sometimes linked to the school meals service
- Day centres, usually run directly by social services departments
- Purchasing laundry services for incontinent people
- Provision of night attendants; only a small proportion of social services departments provide night attendants on anything like an adequate scale
- Welfare facilities for the physically handicapped in general, many of which are particularly relevant to frail old people.

Residential accommodation

Until the early 1980s most residential care for old people was provided in social services-run old people's homes, and very frail elderly people requiring nursing care were looked after in National Health Service (NHS) long-stay hospitals. There have been radical changes in this provision since legislation allowed social services departments to purchase residential rest home and nursing home care in the private sector. In many parts of the United Kingdom this has resulted in a rapid rise in the number of privately owned rest homes and nursing homes, and in some parts of the country – for example, the south coast towns – they are a major industry. On the other hand, some parts of the country have not seen a growth in private sector provision, so, for example, some London boroughs have virtually no private sector provision and continue to rely on social services old people's homes and National Health Service long-stay beds.

The closure of large amounts of National Health Service long-stay capacity with a consequent budgetary shift from health services to social services, has required the generation of criteria, which must be strictly applied, for patients to remain in health service beds once medical treatment has been completed. These criteria vary in different parts of the United Kingdom depending on the pattern of local provision and the size of the private sector.

Generally speaking, very frail elderly patients only remain in NHS long-stay care if they are terminally ill, medically very unstable, or require such intensive nursing care that it would not be reasonable to expect a private sector nursing home to make the necessary provision. Students should find out what the criteria for NHS long-stay care are for their local area.

The whole process for assessment for different levels of residential care is fairly complex and a considerable amount of paperwork is involved. However, broadly speaking, patients who are reasonably independent in the activities of daily living can live in their own homes with support from various statutory services. Those who require help with activities of daily living but do not require nursing care are most suitably placed in rest homes, while those who do require nursing care, particularly if they are immobile, would be eligible for a nursing home unless they fulfil the above-mentioned criteria for health service long-stay care.

Sheltered accommodation

There is no standard pattern for sheltered housing. Often it consists of a cluster of bungalows or low-rise flats occupied only by old people and in a quiet neighbourhood but near shops. Recent purpose-built blocks of flatlets, for either single or married people, are often of excellent quality and include a restaurant and communal sitting rooms in the complex.

Some such developments have been provided by local authorities and some by private organizations specializing in the provision of housing for elderly people. Many of these sheltered units are supervised by a warden whose duty is confined to daily checks that all is well with the residents, either through an intercom or by personal visit, and to help when needed; the warden's duties do not include shopping, domestic cleaning or personal services.

Residents in this type of accommodation must be reasonably self-sufficient, and able to cook, clean and care for themselves to some extent, but they will very often depend heavily on the support of home help services. They are also eligible for any other statutory help which can be provided to people living in their own homes.

The home help service

The home help service is a powerful prop for many old people. Most home helps work part-time and live in the community they serve.

The tasks undertaken by home helps vary from authority to authority but most will include washing up, shopping and bed-making, general tidying and making sure that doors and windows are secure. Some home help services also provide cleaning and help with cooking and washing. Home help services are provided directly by some social services departments, and in other districts are purchased by social services from private home help organizations.

Home helps also provide company for lonely old people and a warm personal relationship is often established between an old person and the home help, whose arrival may be the only social event of the day. The service is charged to the old person, but this is dependent upon an old person's means. Clearly, the cost depends upon the length and frequency of the sessions given. Typically, an old person will have a home help 2 or 3 times a week for about an hour, but in some cases a 7-day-a-week service is required.

'Meals on wheels'

This is an important service which enables frail old people living at home to receive prepared food regularly. The pattern of the provision varies.

In some districts a great deal of support is given by voluntary organizations such as the Red Cross and Age Concern. Some social services departments provide 'meals on wheels' directly from their own facilities and some purchase the service from private companies or give financial support to voluntary services.

The frequency of provision of 'meals on wheels' to an individual will depend on preference and need. Some only require one or two meals weekly, though many opt to receive 'meals on wheels' five or even seven times per week. A charge is made for the meal, and since there is no statutory duty to provide 'meals on wheels', the charge made reflects the cost of production and delivery. In some parts of the country, private 'meals on wheels' companies are able to supply more sophisticated home delivery meals to those who can afford to purchase them.

Day Centres

Day centres are not part of the hospital service but are really clubs for old people. They provide meals, some kind of recreational activity and an opportunity for an old person to meet others. Arrangements for attendance are made by hospitals, family doctors or social workers.

Separate day centres are mostly found in large towns, and in some smaller communities day centres are sometimes provided in local authority old people's homes.

A number of voluntary organizations, including churches and Age Concern, run day centres in some parts of the country. Loneliness being as prevalent as it is amongst old people, the day centres perform a useful function. They are not, however, a place for management of the physically sick. This is the role of the day hospital, which conversely is not intended for use as a club.

Incontinence service

The initial assessment, diagnosis and management plan for incontinent patients is the responsibility of the health services. The service is often coordinated by district nurses, who cooperate with specialist continence nurses based in hospitals. Ideally, an incontinence clinic, run by a geriatrician with a special interest in incontinence, should be available to investigate patients in whom the cause of incontinence is not clear.

On the other hand, some social services departments provide a service for incontinent patients and their relatives in which soiled bed linen is taken away and returned clean. A charge is made to the patient to cover costs.

Night attendants

This service provides someone (who is not usually a nurse) to look after infirm old people during the evening or through the night. The main aim is to relieve the burden on caring relatives and give them a night off. This is not a statutory service and provision varies from one part of the country to another. The cost is charged to the old person.

Care of the dying

Medical education and practice rightly lay great emphasis on the preservation of life. The student must learn and the physician must realize, however, that because a medical or surgical procedure is possible, it is not necessarily right and the doctor who cannot see that there is a human being inside a tangle of clinical problems is not the person to look after dying patients. It is important, therefore, that the emphasis on preservation of life should not blunt the doctor's sensitivity to care of dying people and particularly should not make the physician see death as a failure. This unconscious feeling may impose a barrier between the doctor and the sympathetic care of a dying patient. There is a danger that the physician may feel there is nothing to offer, and being embarrassed, may quickly pass by the bed of the terminally ill patient. Some doctors also rationalize this feeling by suggesting that the patient is unable to bear the truth. The result of all this may be that contacts between the doctor and patient centre on trivialities and untruths and prevent the dying patient from obtaining the help and support which might be expected from the physician.

In many ways, death in old age is of a different quality to the death of younger people.

The majority of people dying in old age have come to terms with the fact that life is finite, and are prepared to die. Death in younger people often seems more unjust and may be more of a tragedy for those who are left behind.

The following discussion is not concerned exclusively with death in old age. The management of dying patients and care of their relatives is an important part of the education of all doctors.

In countries with advanced health-care systems the majority of people live into old age. Consequently, there is no doubt that the experience of close contact with a dying person is no longer universal in the first half of most people's lives. Consequently, children and young people are less likely to experience the understanding of death and of bereavement which can only come from personal involvement. Many people have reached middle age without having any first-hand experience of death whatsoever.

Furthermore, the facts that about 75% of deaths in Britain and North America occur in hospital and that bodies are laid out in funeral parlours rather than in people's homes are other changes in the behaviour of our society which keep death a remote experience. In the 1980s and 1990s there has been an increasing awareness amongst doctors and nurses of the important role which they may play in relation to death and dying and there are many excellent examples of good practice throughout the United Kingdom, not only in specialist units dealing with dying patients, but also on ordinary medical and surgical wards and in acute geriatric units.

The mental aspects of dying

An American psychiatrist, Dr Elizabeth Kubler-Ross, in her book on death and dying divides the dying process into five stages:

- *The stage of denial*. This is the first stage 'No, not me, it cannot be true.' Dr Kubler-Ross believes this is an almost universal reaction and emphasizes how important it is for doctors and nurses to respect the patient's wishes in allowing this stage to continue as long as may be required: a period which may vary from a few hours to many months. It will pass and will be replaced by partial acceptance.

- *The stage of anger*. This is the second stage: 'Why me?' This anger may be projected to members of staff and the patient's family. It is a difficult stage to handle and it is important that the attendant should understand the reason for the anger and not take it personally.

- *The stage of bargaining*. The fact is accepted, but the patient tries to obtain certain promises, from God or from the staff, perhaps. For example, a patient may ask to be allowed to live long enough to attend a daughter's wedding, although the real objective is to prolong life. These promises may be associated with guilt and the doctor should not brush them aside lightly.

- *The stage of depression*. The depression may be two-fold, partly induced by loss suffered already, as a result of mastectomy or hysterectomy, for instance, but more importantly by the losses which are pending. This depression may be suffered silently and patients should be encouraged to express their sorrow and certainly not told to 'look on the bright side'.

- *The stage of acceptance*. This is the final stage and it is particularly important that this should not be disturbed by ill-advised, last-ditch surgical procedures or chemotherapy attempting to snatch a few more weeks of life. The period of acceptance leading to death is one characterized by sleep and a diminished wish for verbal communication. It should not be mistaken for a happy stage. It is a stage almost devoid of feelings. The patient wishes to be left alone more and it is the family who now increasingly require the doctor's support.

All those who are especially involved in the care of dying patients emphasize that the doctor's role in relation to these mental attributes is to be prepared to listen, to share realities with the patient whenever possible and not to make abrupt statements about prognosis. In particular, patients should never be told that they have 'x' number of months or years to live. If doctors will listen they can usually guide their patients into a real acceptance of their situation without either maintaining an unreal charade on the one hand or being unfeelingly brusque on the other.

Patients often pick up clues about their real situation from all that is going on around them. If they wish to talk about these things the doctors and nurses should make time to listen to them. At the very end a physical presence for a little while, a period of nonverbal communication, is what is needed and reassurances can be conveyed by facial expression and hand pressure.

While most dying patients wish to come to a realization of their situation, albeit in their own time, most will also wish to cling to some vestige of hope, however unreal. In such circumstances, therefore, the doctors should make it quite clear that while there is nothing else that can be done to remove the pathological process, everything possible will continue to be done to relieve symptoms and prevent distress.

Physical attributes

In old age, dying is frequently preceded by immobility, incontinence and mental abnormality. In one survey it was found that 40% of people over 65 had one or more of these three disabilities lasting for a month prior to death and 20% had one or more of them lasting for a year prior to death.

In any country, as a population becomes more aged, and the proportion of people in the over-80 age group grows, these types of problem become an increasing feature of the terminal care of people who are dying. Of course, this indicates the burden which has to be carried by relatives and these are important reasons why old people are often admitted to hospital or to nursing homes for their period of dying. It is particularly important to identify symptoms of physical discomfort such as pain, respiratory distress, nausea and vomiting. The control of pain is a paramount responsibility and the armamentarium of analgesic drugs now available will allow this to be done with complete effectiveness in the majority of cases. Occasionally intractable pain requires a neurosurgical approach to cut the pain-carrying tracts within the spinal cord.

Control of pain

It is important to select an adequate analgesic. It is the doctor's responsibility to ensure that consecutive doses are given to anticipate the recurrence of pain.

Analgesics should not be given mechanically on a timed basis unless this is giving good control of the pain. It is bad practice when patients have to wait in pain until the next dose is due. Therefore, the correct dose and timing interval has to be tailored to each individual patient. Indeed, by such means the total amount of analgesic needed in the long run is often less than with rigidly timed or haphazard administration. It should be emphasized once again that the distress of pain in dying should no longer be suffered by patients.

Simple analgesics should be used to begin with including paracetamol, dihydrocodeine and nonsteroidal anti-inflammatory drugs, depending on the nature and cause of the pain. If those fail to control pain properly, opiates should be introduced. If the patient is able to swallow, morphine can be given by mouth, either in normal solution or slow-release form. If swallowing is not possible, diamorphine can be given by injection, either intermittently or by continuous infusion. The dose required needs to be 'titrated' against the pain control, and in some cases patients can be responsible for regulating the speed of infusion themselves.

There is no advantage to giving diamorphine by mouth since it is hydrolysed to morphine at gut level. Pain control is often potentiated by giving a small dose of a tranquillizer such as haloperidol or thioridazine to diminish anxiety. Pain may of course be due to complications such as pneumonia, a pathological fracture or a urinary infection. The use of surgery or antibiotics may be indicated in these cases to relieve the pain. If powerful pain control is required with little or no sedation, the selective synthetic opiate tramadol is very useful.

It is important to control nausea and vomiting, and drugs such as cyclizine, prochlorperazine and metacClopramide are useful. Domperidone is also very helpful, and less sedating than the phenothiazine derivatives. Some patients with severe nausea associated with chemotherapy are best treated with specific serotonin antagonists such as ondansetron and tropisetron.

Severe respiratory distress can be difficult to control. If the patient is hypoxic, oxygen replacement therapy can give some relief, though it is often necessary to use major narcotics such as diamorphine to control severe terminal breathlessness, and troublesome respiratory tract secretions can be reduced with hyoscine.

Where to die

In the United Kingdom the majority of patients die in hospital or in a nursing home. There has been an increasing tendency to refer very frail elderly people to hospital, sometimes inappropriately. The reasons for this trend are not entirely clear, though there seems to be a steadily increasing expectation that hospital services will take over the management of this final phase of a patient's life. It is probably true that many old people would prefer to die at home if facilities were available for their care and if they did not feel they were being a burden to their relatives. Whenever possible, therefore, domiciliary services should be mobilized to make it possible for the dying person to stay in familiar surroundings where individual personal needs are much more likely to be acceded to.

In hospital, patients may be admitted to any of a whole variety of wards and it is probably best that those who have had investigations and treatment in a surgical or medical ward and have come to know and trust the staff should be readmitted to that ward should hospitalization be necessary at the end of their lives.

A number of special hospitals or hospices for the care of dying patients have been created throughout the United Kingdom and in many other countries, some by religious organizations and some secular. They usually attempt to admit patients only for the very end stages of their terminal care, and often organize domiciliary services for support at home up to that point. These hospitals or hospices for the dying are not the forbidding places which they may sound, since they are usually bright and sunny and staffed by doctors and nurses who are specially skilled in the management of dying patients. The staff are trained to listen and they are experts in the pharmacological management of dying. They aim to involve the family from the beginning and their success is apparent to all who have had contact with them.

The question that arises is to what extent special hospices and hospitals for the dying should be created, and to what extent good practice in the care of terminally ill people should be part and parcel of the responsibility of general hospitals. There is no doubt that the hospices have acted as centres of excellence, used for teaching as well as for care, and have greatly influenced the way in which dying patients are managed in general hospitals and in private sector nursing homes.

Bereavement

Care of the dying inevitably moves to care of the bereaved and there is great advantage if continuity of care can be maintained for both the dying patient and the surviving relatives. Bereavement is a period of grieving and the expression of grief would seem to be an essential process for the bereaved. Doctors should see, therefore, that bereaved relatives have the opportunity to go through the stages of the process of grieving. These are likely to be at first a stage of numbness, followed by weeping and sobbing and then a stage of depression. It is generally best to allow the bereaved to live through these stages and not to try and short-circuit them unless they appear interminable.

In old age the depression following bereavement may not be self-limiting and there is, therefore, a time when treatment may be needed. This may involve simple encouragement to socialize or it may require treatment with antidepressant drugs or psychiatric management.

On the death of a spouse an old person may find the loss of pension means that he or she is less well off and important decisions may have to be taken about whether to remain alone, move in with relatives or apply for some other form of care. These decisions should not be taken precipitately and certainly not within the first few weeks of bereavement. No irrevocable decisions of this type should be made until the main period of grieving has passed.

Euthanasia

Euthanasia is a topic of public discussion in a number of countries, and has been the subject of parliamentary bills in the United Kingdom, although these have not been successful and euthanasia is illegal in Britain.

This is the state of affairs in most countries, though Australia has now made special provision for euthanasia under very strictly controlled circumstances and euthanasia is likely to be decriminalized in Holland. Therefore, it is important that doctors should know what is meant by euthanasia and consider its implications since they will almost certainly be asked to express an opinion about it from time to time.

The first important matter is to consider a definition of euthanasia. This may be best understood as the deliberate termination of life under carefully defined conditions, with legal agreement, being carried out in the presence of witnesses and with the agreement of the patient and relatives. The essential element, however, is that of request and euthanasia has been defined by some authors as 'homicide upon request'. It must be distinguished from suicide, which is not illegal, from assisted suicide, which is a crime, and from other methods of life termination which can be described as senicide or dementicide: that is, the killing of aged and demented people respectively. None of these is what is understood as euthanasia and all are criminal acts.

It should be emphasized also that euthanasia is not the acceleration of death as a result of side-effects of drugs used for the relief of intractable pain, for in this case the drug is used with the intention of treating pain. Nor is it about the deliberate withholding of an antibiotic or other technical or surgical procedures which might have the effect of temporarily prolonging a dying patient's life. It must be understood that euthanasia is the bringing about of a patient's death at his or her request.

In the United Kingdom there is relatively little support amongst doctors for the legalization of euthanasia, though there are some signs that this is gradually changing and some British doctors are known to be sympathetic towards the Australian position on this issue. The most basic reasons for objecting to euthanasia are on moral grounds, but it is worth recalling that euthanasia has a number of practical implications as well: for instance, there are the interests of the patient's relatives who in an emotionally charged situation are likely to have ambivalent feelings of attachment and of wanting to be free, and who may also have material and financial interests relating to the patient's death.

Of equal or perhaps greater importance would be the breach of trust likely to be created between patients and physician or nurse which could be perceived by other very ill people as a potential threat, particularly those who do not understand the legal arguments surrounding euthanasia.

26

Some legal aspects of geriatric care

The content of this chapter pertains to the law pre-vailing in England and Wales. The position will be similar in most countries, though students are advised to take steps to find out how the law in their own country varies with respect to the legal arrangements for elderly people unable to direct their own affairs.

Patients unable to manage their own affairs

It must be emphasized that patients who are men-tally clear, with no evidence or minimal evidence of cognitive impairment, remain in charge of their own affairs and destiny, and this legal status must be respected by health care and social services professionals. For example, it often transpires that a frail elderly person insists on returning home from hospital after a period of treatment, even though the professional staff in hospital are of the opinion that the patient will be at substantial physical risk. In these circumstances the patient's wish must be respected and every effort must be made to provide services to support that patient at home.

However, it is a different matter when an elderly patient is suffering from significant cognitive impairment, for example, due to Alzheimer's dis-ease or vascular dementia, because in such a case it will be necessary for other people to take charge of the patient's affairs. Of course, it is essential that any potentially reversible pathology is dealt with before the patient is deemed to be permanently incapable of making the right decisions. In such cir-cumstances there are a number of possible ways forward, as outlined below:

- If the patient is terminally ill there is no need to take urgent steps to appoint an individual with power of attorney over the patient's affairs because the patient's death is anticipated in the near future.
- The patient may have taken the necessary legal steps, whilst still mentally capable of doing so, to hand over the running of his or her affairs to another individual by signing the legal documents transferring power of attorney. Under such circumstances the person holding the power of attorney can make decisions on, for example, financial matters on the patient's behalf.
- If the patient does not own substantial property and lives in accommodation rented from a local authority or from a private person, the social services department will first ask the medical attendant in hospital to certify in writing that the patient is unable to manage his or her affairs, is very unlikely to return to the rented accommodation and that it would be in the patient's best interests for the tenancy to be terminated and the effects sold. The action required will be taken by a relative if one can be found who is willing to do so. If none can be found, the social services department will make the arrangements. Money from the sale of the patient's property or goods will be paid to the patient.
- If the patient has substantial property, such as ownership of a house, investments, incoming rent, private pensions and trusts etc., the matter is more complicated and it will be necessary to apply to the Court of Protection for appointment of an individual with power of attorney over the patient's affairs.

The Court of Protection

This exists specifically to protect and control the administration of the property and affairs of persons who, through mental disorder, are incapable of managing their own affairs. This work applies to people of all ages, but is of special relevance to old people because of their high prevalence of mental confusion.

The Court is not a court in the ordinary sense of the word but the title of an office; its address is Staffordshire House, 25 Store Street, London. The Court will consider taking over the administration of a patient's affairs only if a properly completed originating application is made to it. The originating application is almost always drawn up and submitted by a solicitor, usually under instruction from a relative, or by the legal branch of a local authority. Personal applications can, however, be made directly to the Court and the official solicitor of the Court can also originate an application.

The person in whose name the originating application is made is almost always the nearest of the relatives if there are any. This should be the husband or wife, if alive; and if the spouse is alive but does not originate the application, a reason has to be given. If there is no spouse, the nearest relative can choose to originate, and in the event of there being no relatives, a friend or even a creditor or debtor may apply. If there is conflict about the best originator, the court will choose; the nearest of kin will be preferred, or the person most likely to bring out the whole truth.

The patient's hospital doctor will be involved in this originating application only to the extent of being required, on request, to provide for the purpose either a medical affidavit on the Court's form CP2 for ordinary cases, or a medical certificate form CP3 in small property cases. This form requests information on the medical reasons why a patient is believed incapable of managing his or her affairs, whether the surroundings can be appreciated etc. In cases of gross dementia the evidence is usually plentiful and unequivocal, but there may be real doubt, in which case the doctor is wise to get the support of a senior colleague experienced in such decisions, or the opinion of a psychiatrist.

The papers, including the doctor's affidavit or certificate, are seen by the Court and the next step is that the patient is served with notice of originating proceedings. The Court can dispense with service of this notice if it is satisfied that the patient is incapable of understanding a notice, but it rarely does so. The notice must be seen by the patient without delay. Proof that he or she has been served with the notice usually falls to the lot of the hospital doctor, who is required to complete form CP7 certifying that the patient has seen the notice. This may entail futile attempts to explain the legal document to a profoundly demented or aphasic patient who clearly cannot comprehend it at all. The simplest way is to explain the state of affairs on form CP7. The patient has, however, a legal right to object within 7 days in writing only to the Court, either directly or by instructing a solicitor. The patient can contest the view that he or she is not fit to manage his or her affairs and can object to the proposed receiver, or give a view of how the property should be managed.

On receiving the objection the Court may:

1. make no order; that is, the Court will not be involved
2. proceed with the order on the Master's (senior administrator's) discretion, if the patient seems unequivocally unable to manage his or her affairs
3. if there is doubt, the Master will ask for the Lord Chancellor's medical visitors to report on the patient's mental condition and advise on capability.

If there is no objection and the proceedings continue, the Court will appoint a receiver, but this and subsequent management do not involve the medical attendant.

The Court of Protection should not be confused with power of attorney in which a person of sound mind voluntarily gives to someone else legal responsibility for the management of his or her financial affairs and estate, either generally or for some specific act.

Patients admitted under an order for their own care and protection

It happens, fortunately rarely, that a patient with gross physical or mental disease is believed by a medical attendant, either the family doctor or hospital doctor, to be in imperative need of hospital treatment because either the patient's own life or the life and health of others will otherwise be threatened. The patient may, however, refuse to cooperate. Admission to hospital or other public institution can then be compelled through Section 47 of the *Public Assistance Act* (1947) by an order of a magistrate's court made on evidence submitted to the local health authority, with the advice of the district community physician, to whom the family doctor or hospital doctor should first apply with an account of the case.

Where old people are concerned, the type of patient involved is often a recluse, living alone in squalid conditions and sometimes suffering from malnutrition or a disabling physical condition. Almost always there is a large mental element, though this will often not amount to a frank psychosis.

Senile breakdown in standards of hygiene and cleanliness is a syndrome which often raises the possibility of compulsory admission of an old person. Often neighbours will indignantly demand the patient's removal, fearful for their own safety and on occasion with good reason, since some socially isolated people are accident-prone, especially where fire is concerned. The order lasts 48 hours only, but can be renewed. Sometimes a brief period of treatment and rehabilitation is enough to allow the patient to go home, especially if it is possible to go to live with relatives, but often removal to hospital will permanently shatter the patient's ability to survive, however unsatisfactorily, in the community. For this reason, compulsory admission under Section 47 should be avoided whenever possible.

Old age abuse

It has become clear through research in the United Kingdom and a number of other countries that elderly people are sometimes subjected to a variety of forms of abuse, usually by younger relatives. This may take the form of actual physical assault (though this is quite rare), verbal abuse, physical and social neglect, and financial abuse.

Physical assault in these circumstances usually takes the form of rough and impatient handling, often by an otherwise caring relative who has become exhausted and exasperated by the continual burden of looking after a very frail elderly person. In extreme cases of physical assault, it would be necessary to involve the police, though much can be done to alleviate the problem by providing proper support for caring relatives. The other forms of abuse are more difficult to detect and prove, though tactful questioning by a well-trained social worker will often help to gain an idea of the extent of the problem. Occasionally the staff of residential homes, nursing homes or hospitals are implicated in old age abuse of one sort or another, in which case it may be necessary to take appropriate disciplinary action or involve the licensing authorities or police.

Further reading

Andrews K 1991 Rehabilitation of the older adult. Arnold, London

Brocklehurst JC, Tallis RC, Fillit HM (eds) 1992 Textbook of Geriatric Medicine, 4th edn. Churchill Livingstone, Edinburgh

Evans JG, Williams TF (eds) 1992 Oxford textbook of geriatric medicine. Oxford University Press, Oxford

Hall MRP, MacLennan WJ, Lye MDW 1993 Medical care of the elderly, 3rd edn. John Wiley and Sons, Chichester

Holliday R 1995 Understanding Ageing. Cambridge University Press, Cambridge

Kamal A, Brocklehurst JC 1991 A colour atlas of geriatric medicine, 2nd edn. Mosby-Wolfe, London

Overstall PW 1997 Ageing and disease. In: Souhami RL, Moxham J (eds) Textbook of medicine, 3rd edn. Churchill Livingstone, Edinburgh, ch 9, p 155

MacLennan WJ 1995 Principles of geriatric medicine. In: Edwards CRW et al (eds) Davidson's Principles and practice of medicine, 17th edn, Churchill Livingstone, Edinburgh, ch 17, p 1117

Pathy MSJ (ed) 1991 Principles and practice of geriatric medicine, 2nd edn. John Wiley and Sons, Chichester

Shukla RB, Brooks D (eds) 1996 A guide to care of the elderly. The Stationery Office Publications, London

Journals

Age and Ageing
Journal of the American Geriatric Society
Geriatric Medicine

This list is by no means comprehensive but represents examples of the range of literature available in the field of geriatric medicine.

Index